MALE INFERTILITY

FIGHTING BACK

MALE INFERTILITY

FIGHTING BACK

by

Belinda Barnes

FORESIGHT

The Association for the Promotion of Preconceptual Care

All profits from the sale of this book go to the FORESIGHT Charity.

ISBN 0-9545933-2-4

Typeset by Karen Robertson

Origination and Production by
Print-Rite, 31 Parklands, Freeland, Oxon OX29 8HX

Published by
FORESIGHT
The Association for the Promotion of Preconceptual Care
28 The Paddock
Godalming
Surrey
GU7 1XD

Registered Charity No 279160

CONTENTS

PREFACE

by Dr Sarah Temple

When I met Belinda Barnes I was attempting to conceive my first child, Charlie. I had had a late miscarriage eighteen months previously, had a diagnosis of endometriosis and an appointment pending at an Infertility Clinic. I am convinced that attention to diet and other lifestyle factors, together with complementary therapies and relaxation techniques played a significant part in my husband and I becoming healthier, feeling fitter and happier together. We were fortunate not to need any medical intervention - but enhanced well being is of value for everyone - including those undergoing IVF. We now have two beautiful boys- Charlie and Douglas.

In my work as a GP, I frequently see couples struggling to come to terms with infertility. Stories are many and varied - but almost universally considerable strain is put on relationships. Attention to well being can enable couples to regain a sense of physical and emotional balance.

Belinda's latest contribution to The Foresight Programme offers yet more practical advice to couples seeking to optimise pre-conception care as well as tackling one of the most difficult areas of all - male infertility. Based on over twenty years working with infertile couples she explores the affects of lifestyle factors such as diet, smoking, alcohol, environmental toxins and electromagnetics. Stress and anxiety are acknowledged as interfering with both immunological function and hormonal balance.

The holistic approach integrates conventional medical screening and treatment with lifestyle changes and complementary therapies. Belinda brings these together in a readable and practical form.

Dr Sarah Temple MA, MBBChir MRCGP DRCOG

MALE INFERTILITY

CHAPTER 1

WHERE ARE WE AT?

There is no greater tragedy the world can hold than infertility. Death can be harshly cruel in separating too soon, but within the grief there is memory, and in memory lives what has been. In infertility there is only longing, and the pain is the greater because only those involved cry internally as the world passes by. There is no funeral, no hymns, no flowers, no mourning, yet every month there seems to be a funeral of dreams as once again the son or daughter, who would have been so loved, is not on the way. The clock of life ticks relentlessly on, and the fear that they may never join us is harder and harder to hold at bay.

So you too have a fertility problem? You and one in six of all the couples in the United Kingdom. We need to find out exactly why, and we need to correct this and overcome it. The FORESIGHT programme is often the best way towards this with a success rate of 66.2% with those who come to us with male infertility and follow the programme faithfully.

Present day infertility is not an isolated problem. It is part of a greater scene. Carlson et al in 1992 noted evidence for a decreased quality of sperm over the previous forty years. The deterioration of human sperm is following an evident trend in ever decreasing standards of physical and mental health in all species.

As a result, at least in part, of widespread toxic pollution of air and water, many species in the wild are also under threat from the inability to reproduce. In the rivers, as a result of pesticides and detergents and other chemicals from factory effluent that are contaminating their living space, combining to form xeno-estrogens, fish are becoming hermaphrodite and are unable to reproduce. Pesticides used in modern farming are hugely reducing the insect population, so by using these we are creating a food shortage for birds, which is compromising their reproduction. Many species of butterflies have been destroyed and can never be regained. Many different species of wild flowers are also gone forever as the result of herbicide spraying. If we count the population of any wild species at all, we find it is dwindling away. What is toxic to one species is toxic to all. We are all a part of an inter-dependant whole.

So, in the human arena are we becoming healthier and more vital? *We are not.*

The air and water is more poisoned, while the nutrients that defend the integrity of the body are present in smaller amounts than formerly in much of the food we eat. This disturbs a vital balance between positive and negative influences in the body.

The damage to the basic integrity of the whole organism affects the testicle and the ovary. It also affects every other organ and cell in the body, including the brain. Each human cell can only take so much.

Conversely, this is why we find that when we can restore the basic health of the whole body, we can also, in almost all cases, restore the natural fertility.

Let us look at what has been happening.

Physical and Mental Deterioration

Professor Rimland, of California, who has been testing the IQ of United States boys applying to enter the Army over many years, has noticed a discreet but continuing drop in the IQ scores of those coming forward. He has calculated that the average IQ score *deteriorates by one point per year.* Nothing much to worry about in any one year perhaps - *but over twenty years?*

Then we find the examination standards world-wide have been lowered to accommodate the lowered academic performance. This may temporarily mask an embarrassing social disaster, but is anybody enquiring WHY this is necessary? Surely it would be expected that standards of intelligence will advance rather than regress?

We need to take stock. It matters. *The whole panoramic scene tends to deteriorate in unison.* Divorce, crime, perversion, suicide and murder are all on the increase. Degenerative illness, allergy, mental illness and "learning difficulties" are nearly swamping the NHS and the Department of Education. Children of mothers who lack appropriate maternal responses are being increasingly dumped all day into nurseries at a more and more tender age. Chronic illness such as asthma and eczema, and atypical brain development leading to dyslexia, dysgraphia, hyperactivity and AHDD plague the schools. Too many teenagers are turning to drugs and alcohol to prop up sick minds and bodies. This, of course, makes them sicker!

The Arts

In the arts, so called "modern art" is a daub or a pile of bricks; so called "modern music" is a discordant noise. Some leading figures in the art world and professional musicians try to pretend otherwise, as their livelihood hinges on maintaining public interest, but few normal citizens are fooled. Too often the "modern novel" is sadism, cynicism or "soft porn". Too many modern films and television writers give us plays that tend to be nothing but repetitious scenes of debauchery and smashing people to pieces with a blunt instrument. (Twenty years ago it seemed nothing but car chases and boys dodging around packing cases, cars or buildings with a gun; now the "heroes" corner the quarry and batter him to death.)

Mental Function

Both mental function and fertility are very closely linked to the general health.

If the body is stressed by nutritional deficiencies as the result of poor food, by high levels of toxins, by the xeno-estrogens, by chemical effluent, narcotics and heavy metals in the surrounding environment, or by the invasion of bugs and viruses, *no part of the body will function well.* This includes the brain and the thought processes; *and the testicle and sperm-making equipment therein.*

This is why it is imperative you improve your long-term general health. Fertility was designed to complement strength, virility, and competence. You need to be around to protect, provide for and guide your little person that you are creating; you do not want to be fading at an early stage once you are into family life.

You are thinking fighting fit! Ready for walking up and down the bedroom at 2.00am, when she-who-did-the-birth-bit is in need of her sleep. We are talking about a delighted and congratulatory mode when someone calls out at 6.00am that they want their potty. We are talking about cricket on the lawn at the end of a long day's work, played with someone who is going to challenge your decision as to whether he was out or not. We are not talking Soft Options here!

To return to our original starting point and the reason you bought this book; one man in eleven is infertile. The health of the modern testicle has deteriorated so that very frequently indeed it can no longer produce enough viable and purposeful sperm.

However the good news is, on a personal level, in almost every case, this can be rectified in a matter of months. On a national scale, this whole disaster scenario needs to be tackled radically; so we can all have a much better life. On a planetary scale, it is imperative that it is tackled, or ultimately this is goodbye to the human race!

So, what do we do? Well, recent FORESIGHT work has shown that at least 66.2% of men with a long-term fertility problem recovered and successfully fathered children on the full FORESIGHT programme. Details of the Study can be found later in the book.

It is interesting to note that the progression towards success increases quite dramatically with the commitment given to the programme. In the recent count-up of people coming to us with male infertility we found that the success rate was:

No part in FORESIGHT	A Small Part	Most Of It	All Of It
16.2%	21.3%	27.8%	66.2%

It is also worth noting that those who did nothing at all were close to the Human Fertility and Embryology Authority's average figure for "high-tech" success (22.6%). Some IVF units achieve even less than this.

Our suggestion would be to follow the FORESIGHT programme carefully for at least a year, as, going on these figures, it is likely that at least 2 out of every 3 of you will achieve a baby without further ado or expense

- while at the same time enhancing your basic health, and the health and mental ability of your future baby.

If at first you don't succeed . . . then there are a whole range of practitioners with all manner of alternative skills at their fingertips.

FORESIGHT is here to help you to complete the first stage, and can help you find alternative practitioners in your area if you should need or wish to move on to the second stage. Do not be down-hearted. Onward!

A Brief Summary of The FORESIGHT Programme for Male Infertility

Our main areas of concern include:

1 Eating healthy organic food

The avoidance of food contaminants such as pesticides, harmful bacteria and hazardous food additives. Food choices for nutritional value. Filtering the drinking water. Keep to organic foods as much as you can and leave out refined carbohydrates (white flour, bread, rice etc and white sugar).

Glance down the foods on page 80 to 82 for the most rich in nutrients. A good rotation round the week for the main meal is brown meat, white meat, fish, brown meat, white meat, fish, cheese dish.

One vegetarian dish with cheese, vegetables and whole rice or pasta keeps your hand in for cooking for vegetarian friends!

Get a copy of "Find Out" from FORESIGHT and avoid dangerous additives.

See pages 68 to 89 for organization and further ideas! See also page 86 for menu suggestions.

2 The elimination of smoking, alcohol, street drugs and unnecessary medication.

To break an addiction, try reflexology, acupuncture, homeopathy and hypnotism. All have been found helpful by some people. (Addresses in Appendix IV)

Seize all the help you can get from alternative practitioners (if you find this necessary) but don't smoke and don't drink until the Deed is Done! Whatever it takes, don't weaken!

Just chuck the cigarettes away and focus on the health benefits, and the **money** you save! The latter will amaze you!

See address list at the end of the book for a whole world of help and sympathetic support that is there for you if you need it.

Choose soft non-alcoholic drinks you like before starting to eliminate so there is something there! Avoid those with artificial additives like aspartame. Browse round the fresh juice shelves reading the labels. Waitrose and all the Health Stores have Rice Dream, which is pleasant.

Suggestions: Try a herbal tea for breakfast, plus fresh fruit juice. At work - 11 am de-caf coffee or tea, alcohol-free lager with lunch, tea at teatime. In the evening, a Rice Dream (very nice hot), or de-caf coffee or tea, natural, organic fruit juices galore! Good old fresh water! Wines are now available alcohol free, as is beer! Well, toss it around!

All in a good cause! See also Chapter 4.

3 Genito-urinary and other infections - detection and treatment.

Your nearest large hospital will have a Genito-Urinary Medicine (GUM) Clinic. You do not need a letter of referral. If they do not have a GUM Clinic, they will be able to tell you where the nearest one is.

Check they do all the infections listed on page 119. If they do not, ask them where you can get them done. The more you get checked, the more secure you are. They will need you to give them a blood, urine and semen sample. They will need to test your wife as well. A few days later they will let you know the results. If you are told that an infection is present, then both you and your partner should be treated, either with antibiotics or by homeopathy. See Appendix V for how to find a homeopath. Or, better still contact FORESIGHT for one who is known to them.

After treatment, return to the GUM Clinic for further sampling to make sure the infection has been completely cleared. Occasionally, further treatment is necessary.

4 Allergy, malabsorption and intestinal parasites - detection and treatment.

If you are unsure if you have an allergy, perhaps manifesting as eczema, asthma, depression, migraine, insomnia or similar, for which you have to take frequent or regular medication, or if you suffer from irritable bowel syndrome, this needs help.

Read Chapter 6. If you feel your illness falls into one or more of these categories, study the lists of books, and the contacts for help at the back of this book, and try some common-sense self-help! If things are difficult, find the necessary expertise by contacting FORESIGHT for your nearest practitioner.

Allergies and hypoglycaemia can be banished by dietary manipulation. (This does not necessarily mean having to eat boring food!)

Intestinal parasites can be dealt with in a few weeks by the appropriate antibiotic or homeopathic treatment. Don't be too bashful to ask for help. All of these problems can be conquered in a very few months if approached with a will!

5 Trace element deficiencies and heavy metal toxicities - assessment by hair analysis, interpretation and treatment.

Hair analyses, with programmes for enhancing status to normal levels (essential to fertility and foetal health and development), and cleansing programmes to reduce levels of toxic metals (known to be injurious to sperm and to foetal development) are obtainable through FORESIGHT.

Send FORESIGHT an A5 stamped addressed envelope with a 34p stamp. (NB as of going to press, this is the postage to cover a 100 gram package. Please adjust as appropriate). You will receive a package which contains (amongst other things) the questionnaire and form to send hair for analysis. This tells you how to take the sample and so on.

Please fill in the questionnaire as diligently as possible. This will make the picture clear for us to give help with the interpretation of the hair analysis. Send a hair sample as instructed, and then when you get the results back, follow the suggested vitamin and mineral programme.

Keep in close touch and retest the hair as suggested, as this makes it possible to maximise the help we can give you. The programme we give will be designed to maximise the levels of nutrients that are essential for health and reproductive excellence, and to minimise the level of toxins that interfere with normal sperm development. The work will be part of the ongoing research undertaken by the Charity to further understanding of the causes of infertility, and to overcome it..

6. Environmental factors/Electromagnetism.

You need to eliminate contact with such substances as pesticides, fluoride, mercury amalgams and to stop contact with mobile phones, microwave ovens and other sources of electromagnetic pollution.

Be very wary of using or being close to mobile telephones. The emissions kill sperm and can cause tumours. Avoid cooking things in a microwave. Turn off electric blankets when you get into bed. Turn luminous clocks away from you at night. Limit the use of a VDU to five hours a day maximum.

Be aware of any pylons, mobile phone masts, electric-railways, and so on in your vicinity. If you have any reason to feel you are at risk to electromagnetic pollution, you need to contact Dr Patrick MacManaway or Roy Riggs or Roger Coghill. See Appendix V on page 214 for addresses. They can detect the area of electromagnetic pollution and advise you on a course of action. Eliminating this can encourage sperm development, and guard against chromosomal abnormalities, leukaemia and cancer. A job worth doing.

· · · · · · · · · · · · · · · · · · ·

Read the following chapters for more information on the FORESIGHT programme generally. Firstly, to go into why this programme is necessary, both for conception, and for optimising the future baby's health and development. Secondly, more details on how to do it!

Summary of a Basic Plan of Action for Optimum Sperm Health

The questions we ask regarding optimum health before pregnancy are

A   Is optimising sperm health important?

B   Does it increase fertility in both partners?

C   Does it lessen the chances of miscarriage?

D   Is it vital to prevent malformation?

E   Does it help to prevent prematurity?

F   Will the babies be more likely to achieve a good weight for gestational age?

G   Will preconceptual preparation help to prevent fatigue and post partum depression in the mother?

H   Does it help the mother to prevent pre-eclampsia?

I   Will it promote breast milk?

J   Will the child be happier, healthier and probably more intelligent?

The answer is a resounding YES.

In the following pages we will show how the programme can be followed through. After this, we will go through together what evidence there is that this will be helpful.

Stay on board, this is only the beginning!

CHAPTER 2

THE FORESIGHT SAGA!
THE HISTORY OF FORESIGHT

As you may be wondering where all this is coming from, I think it is appropriate for me to spend a few moments telling you a little bit about the founding of FORESIGHT - the origins of FORESIGHT. (*If this does not interest you at all, skip to Chapter 3!*)

The first thing I must do is to pay tribute to some truly wonderful Americans who helped me at the beginning - (and also to those who are helping us today, Dr Harold Buttram and Dr William Kracht from Quakertown, Pennsylvania, and Dr Allan Liebermann from New England.) In particular at the outset, I learned so much from Dr Elizabeth Lodge-Rees, Dr Carl Pfeiffer, Dr Abe Hoffer, Dr Donald Oberleas, Dr Theron Randolph, and the Englishman, Professor Humphrey Osmond. They were people I knew and talked to personally. I was so fortunate, I received such encouragement, so much knowledge, so much fun and so much practical help. Without them this story would never have been told. Then there were the books of Weston Price, Frank Pottinger, Adelle Davies, Roger Williams, Christopher Norwood, - the list could go on!

FORESIGHT was not invented. It grew. It appeared like an oak tree appears out of an acorn. I will try and share some of this growing period with you, so we will get to know each other better.

In the beginning . . .
I had a hyperactive son. A gluten free diet solved some of his problems, but some were ongoing for very many years. Then I had my daughter and she had two tumours on the spinal cord. This took a lot of resolving, with much terror, anguish, prayer, surgery and with radio therapy. Thank God this was successful. Then my third child was a baby who was so allergic that he could not take any food other than breast milk, even at eight months old, without asthma, eczema and diarrhoea.

By this time you are talking to God very seriously indeed, believe me. Even bargaining. Begging for signs. Asking what to do.

In 1965 the idea came to my husband and me to move out of London. We were looking for clean air, greenery, space and peace. We were lucky enough to move close to two of the most delightful women I have ever met. They were the wife and the sister of Professor Humphrey Osmond, a psychiatrist-with-vision who was at that time working in Canada with Dr Abram Hoffer. He was pioneering the use of nutrients - at that time just supplements of nicotinamide, pyridoxine and vitamin C - with the mentally ill. On his suggestion, I started to give my elder son, then nine years old, nicotinamide - so far as I remember only 20mg a day - and the change was miraculous. Overnight I had a different child. The hyperactivity lessened dramatically. He became able to concentrate and to relate to others. Life at home and at school began to normalise for him (and for us!)

It was ONE turning point.

We had moved next door to a Cheshire Home. I became involved with some of their activities and used to take round surplus vegetables from our garden, so I got to know some people at the Home.

One day in 1973, I had read an article by the playwright Roger MacDougal, who was living in California and who suffered from MS. He had found help from a gluten-free, milk-free diet, and a multivitamin that he had formulated for himself.

I went round and showed the article to the Warden and Matron at the Cheshire Home and explained I knew how to organize a gluten-free diet and would love to help. For some time we were able to help 10 sufferers from MS who we were able to provide with some foods and supplements. All of them made very significant improvements. Some went into complete remission. However the happiness was short-lived.

Unfortunately at the time this was regarded as "unorthodox", and, despite the obvious benefits, it was stopped by the Powers-That-Were. We were not allowed to continue and people regressed. (Although a few years later the idea was taken up again and the approach is now quite widely used.)

At the same time I was in touch with a local Roman Catholic priest who was trying to help people suffering from alcoholism, and with advice from Humphrey Osmond and his colleague, Abe Hoffer, we were able to make abstention much easier for them with detection of allergy, dietary adjustment and supplements. (This endeavour flourished, and some years later, a number of those involved went on to found the Westminster Advisory Centre on Alcoholism).

These three incidents had fully convinced all of us concerned of the relevance of food allergies, and also of vitamin and mineral status, to both physical and mental health.

At this time, I was writing to Humphrey Osmond and Abe Hoffer quite regularly. I joined the associations *Sanity*, the *Schizophrenia Association of Great Britain* and the *McCarrison Society*, to glean all the information I could, also to help to spread the American work to them. Through these organisations I met some doctors in the UK who were into diet, allergies, and so on. Humphrey Osmond came over, also Unabelle Blackwood from Ohio, another mover and shaker, and we gave lunches and meetings for them to meet the English doctors.

My American contacts introduced me to the *Journal of Orthomolecular Psychiatry* and from these pages I met Dr Elizabeth Lodge-Rees, a paediatrician from California. She had written an article on allergy, vitamin and mineral therapy, dyslexia and hyperactivity that seemed to summarise all the knowledge available at that time.

This was another Turning Point.

I wrote to her and said "*Come over to England and have a holiday here! I will take you to stately homes and cathedrals galore if you will tell me all about your work!*" Beth was not a great enthusiast of the stately homes or cathedrals but she came anyway.

I met her at London Airport, and she had brought with her three books - by Weston Price, Frank Pottinger, and Roger Williams. "*I have arms the length of an orang-utang honey, carrying these darned books. You have to look nonchalant or they weigh things and charge you extra.*" I sat up all night reading. Then we talked for a fortnight!

Out in California, she was just starting out on a new enterprise. She had heard that a small piece of hair was taken from the animals in the slaughterhouse and tested to see if they were in good condition. Beth never missed a trick. "*I could do that for my children*" she said.

She and Dr Gary Gordon started their hair analysis laboratory, *Mineralab*, the following year. In 1976 she invited me out to the States to go on a "floating symposium" aboard a ship cruising down the side of Mexico, to learn about mineral metabolism and the reading of mineral analyses. We had Professor Linus Pauling and Dr Virginia Livingstone-Wheeler on board. It was a fabulous nine days of lectures and conversations on the role of minerals in human health. We also made two memorable visits to Mexico (on one occasion getting lost a long way from the quay and nearly missing the boat!)

When I returned to the UK, probably partly because I had been a Nursery Nurse, and partly because people noticed the change in my son, a whole host of people asked me to help with their children with eczema, asthma, dyslexia, diarrhoea, growth retardation, learning difficulties and so on.

I started sending hair samples out to Beth and finding the right supplements for the children in England. Not always easy, as compared with now. Availability of minerals was limited, we had to convert English money into dollars to send samples to the States, and so on.

Like Topsy, it growed. I began to feel strongly, *as I do even more today,* that none of these disastrous health problems should be happening in the first place. It became evident even at that stage that it was all so preventable. It was also noticable that conditions such as eczema and asthma were exacerbated by food additives, pesticides, tetraethyl lead added to petrol etc and that the firms that made these pollutants also made the drugs used to treat the conditions they created.

The next milestone was in 1978. I formed FORESIGHT with five friends, to promote Preconceptual Care, to get things right for the babies from the outset. They were Humphrey Osmond's sister, Dorothy Gale, a midwife, and his wife Jane Osmond, a nurse. Gill Gibbons who worked at the Cheshire Home (and had been involved in all the efforts with MS there), Ruth Jervis, a nutritionist, whose parents founded the health farm, Enton Hall, and Eve Mervyn-Smith, then a Community Health Council Secretary, who thereafter worked with me for over 20 years. Our advisors were Professor John Dickerson, Professor of Human Nutrition at University of Surrey, and Professor Derek Bryce-Smith from the University of Reading who was pioneering work against lead pollution and Dr (later Professor) Philip Barlow of Aston in Birmingham, later of Hull, with seven other natural-health orientated doctors whom I had met mainly through the McCarrison Society.

Our initial intention was modest. It was to gather all the research together, tell them of our positive experiences, work out a possible Plan of Campaign for preconception, so that children need not be born disadvantaged by heavy metal toxicities, allergic illnesses and nutrient deficiencies. We intended to write articles about it. We hoped to interest the media, the medical profession and the Government in the possibilities of the approach. We hoped they would then take over and develop the ideas further.

However, after one article on preconceptual care in the popular press, we were completely inundated by the general public wanting to get more information! We had to write our first booklet very quickly, get it printed at speed and start sending it out!

We found ourselves organising hair analysis in the States for a growing army of people, and the logistics of it became almost overwhelming!

Professor John Dickerson formulated some basic supplements and we asked Cantassium Co., who made for Roger MacDougal, to make them up. (I was still in touch with Roger, who was still helping people with MS.)

So, our original programme was brought into being. We gave advice on sound nutrition, based loosely on the Enton Hall concepts, on hair analysis to optimise mineral status, and we helped people with food allergies to find organisations or doctors who could help them to adjust their lifestyle.

At about the same time, Patrick Halford founded the Institute of Optimum Nutrition. So later, we also started working with nutritionists and other alternative practitioners. We now have a network of 200 people (and growing all the time!) The Committee has gradually altered and grown, and we have a system of local branch secretaries, nationwide.

Another Milestone

Yet another milestone came when, about 2 years into our existence, I was rung by such a lovely woman to ask if our programme would give any help with infertility? She had been trying for 7 years to have a baby.

"I really don't know" I said, *"But I'm game to try, if you are?"*

She and her husband took to the FORESIGHT programme with great enthusiasm, and within a few months, she rang me to tell me she was pregnant.

"What are you hoping for - a boy or a girl?" I asked her.

It was such a sweet reply, *"Would you think it was awfully greedy if I told you I was praying for twins, a boy and a girl? We've waited so long, and I am getting on a bit, this would make it all just perfect!"*

"No, I don't think it's greedy, I think it's eminently sensible. I'll pray too."

About 7 months later, I got this little salmon pink letter. It said: *"Just as we prayed for, John was 5lb 8oz, and Rowina was 4lb 10oz. They are both absolutely beautiful. Thank you so much for praying for us!"*

I stood in the middle of the kitchen floor with this letter, and thought, *"Right, I think I'm meant to do this, then."*

Since then, the infertility work has mounted and mounted and is now about 60% or more of what we do.

In the early days, splendid American researchers came over and stayed with me to give lectures - Humphrey Osmond, Unabelle Blackwood, Beth Lodge-Rees, Carl Pfeiffer, Donald Oberleas, Theron Randolph and David Horrobin, (who was English, but was working in Canada at the time). Beth Lodge-Rees and Carl Pfeiffer and his wife each came several times.

We enlarged the programme a discovery at a time. We learned more about the damage done by the toxic metals from our advisor, Professor Derek Bryce-Smith in the UK, and from Dr Elizabeth Lodge-Rees.

We heard a lot from Arthur and Margaret Wynn about the dangers of smoking and alcohol in pregnancy, and we added smoking and alcohol abstention to the FORESIGHT programme. Margaret and I are still friends - in the spring of 2000 I went to their joint 89th birthday party at the House of Lords! Sadly we have recently lost Arthur - still working until the day he died, aged 91 years. They were a remarkable and wonderful pair, and have made available a great deal of excellent research to the world, by writing very readable books with enticing titles, simplifying for the lay mind a lot of scientific work the ordinary man in the pub would never otherwise be able to access.

Another redoubtable pioneer, Dr Ellen Grant, had been studying the effects of the contraceptive pill on hormone levels and fertility, and from her research, it was clear that the pill does not serve the next generation well. We took her work on board also. Eliminating the use of exogenous hormones and restoring fertility by restoring the natural health, and re-balancing the mineral ratios that have been distorted by these drugs, has become a large part of our work.

We found a delightful Roman Catholic lady, Colleen Norman who is a superb teacher of Natural Family Planning. With her help, replacing pill use with NFP knowledge, (coupled, when people wish, to barrier methods during the fertile phase) has become another mainstay of the FORESIGHT programme.

Dr Ellen Grant also gave us a lot of information on genito-urinary infection. We started testing. A count-up by another doctor found 51 % of women and 47% of men in our population positive (ie having an infection), so we now suggest to all our couples that they check out for GUI on the NHS as a routine part of our programme.

I got to know Mrs Enfys Chapman of PEGS (Pesticides Exposure Group of Sufferers), who had much information on the organophosphate pesticides creating eczema, asthma, diarrhoea etc, as well as destroying fertility. So we have been advocating organically grown food for a very long time - latterly this has become much easier for people, as more organic food is appearing in the supermarkets.

Recently more has become known about parasites. Our nutritionists come forward with new research all the time, and we are now looking much more carefully at irritable bowel syndrome (now about 1 person in 5 of those who contact us, - as you will see from the tables on pages 27 to 28). If in doubt, the Nutritionist arranges a stool test and frequently finds giardia, blastocystic hominus or similar parasites. Coeliac condition, cow's milk allergy or candida are also all quite common.

The charts on the next two pages show the most commonly seen illnesses/conditions of those who have contacted us in the last 4 years. As you will see, most of them are suffering quite a lot with "sub-clinical illnesses". All of this contributes to the reproductive problems. These are, in some cases, directly caused by nutrient deficiencies. In other cases as with the parasites, they actually cause or exacerbate the deficiencies.

The charts show the percentage of people with undiagnosed/untreated/ unresolved illnesses who have contacted FORESIGHT regarding reproductive problems. This may be roughly typical of people with fertility problems nationwide.

Table 1   General Health Problems in Either Partner Contacting FORESIGHT

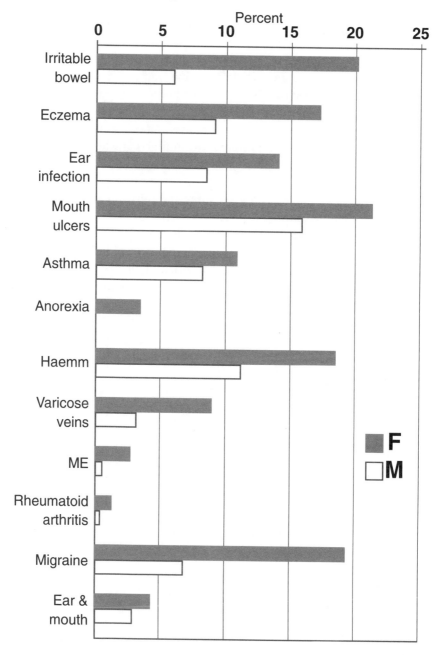

Table 2   Gynaecological Problems in Women Contacting
FORESIGHT

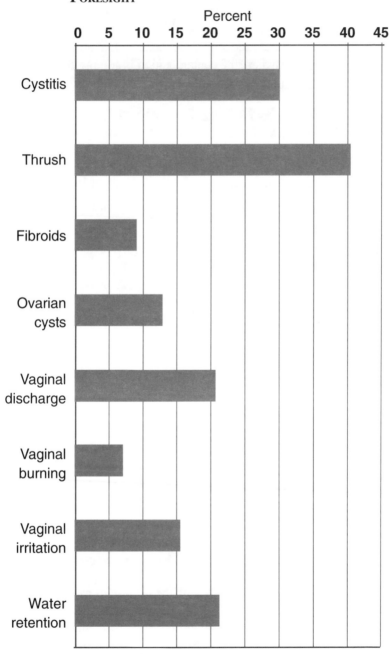

The analysis of hair and the interpretation of the results becomes more sophisticated as we become more experienced. We now have our own laboratory, and formulate our own supplements to more specifically serve the needs of those who come to us. We can now test the water, dust, cosmetics, herbal products etc of those with abnormal levels, so that we can find out where the contamination is coming from, in order to eliminate the source wherever possible. Thus the programme grows and becomes more effective all the time.

During the course of all of this, we have produced four other books. With the help of Gail Bradley, we wrote one for the couples themselves, Planning For A Healthy Baby and one for the health professionals, Preparation for Pregnancy, an Essential Guide. With the late Mrs Vicky Colquhoun I wrote one on hyperactivity, The Hyperactive Child, What The Family Can Do.

Ruth Jervis and her husband wrote the FORESIGHT Wholefood Cookbook. We made a video, Preparing For The Healthier Baby. This is now also on DVD. A Finnish friend, biochemist Tuula Tuormaa, has written a series of very well referenced booklets, summarising the research on all aspects of preconceptual care. We also have an A3 poster which has the full programme on it, and a handful of leaflets on various subjects.

All the above are being updated for our Silver Jubilee this year (2003).

Research Efforts

However, it has been hard to get research off the ground!

In 1982 we tried to do a Study at the University of Aston in Birmingham, but halfway through the Government abolished the Department of the Environment, where our student was working! Dr Philip Barlow who had been running it, went to the University of Hull, and our student went off to find a much better paid job!

A year later we tried to do a study with the Cranfield Institute of Social Studies, but our financial resources were small and our Researcher fell on hard times, and told us she had to find better paid employment, and left us!

Somewhat chagrined and dismayed we put what little hard-won funds we had in hand towards a cash-needy study by Professor Bryce-Smith and Dr Neil Ward. They were studying minerals in the placental tissue, and the correlation with effects on the babies.

Dr Ward told me they also needed help with ferrying the placental tissue down from St George's Hospital to their base at Ascot. I volunteered to drive it down. *Never do that!*

I will simply say that the samples were inadequately wrapped. So, late afternoon saw me freaking out in the driveway at Ascot. This was my first meeting with Neil Ward.

"Come away Mrs Barnes" he said, "come away. We have students to cope with situations like this. They will spring clean your car, while you and I have a cup of tea a long way away from this."

This proved to be another milestone.

This cup of tea started a long and happy relationship with Surrey University where Neil was just about to take up a new post. We worked with them for 9 years with a series of three students to study our work and put things together. In 1990 we fundraised for, and, with the help of Mr and Mrs Chapman of PEGS, got them an Inductively Coupled Plasma-Mass Spectrometer (ICPMS) and they took over the hair analysis.

The last period of 1990-92 produced the small study of 367 couples who gave birth to 327 healthy babies, with only one low birthweight baby who was 5lb 3oz, details of which are given on pages 31 to 32. However, in the end, the volume of work FORESIGHT generated was swamping them! We had to get together our own laboratory. This was a very major exercise, which depleted our financial resources, and took a long time to get off the ground. Nonetheless, the Laboratory is now up and running with our excellent Lab Director, Michael Cain, and we are doing a steady stream of hair analyses and other relevant work.

Another Turning Point

The year after we took over the laboratory work, Cantassium/Larkhill Green Farm sold out, so we had to take over the manufacture of our own supplements. We hope FORESIGHT will now be on a sounder financial footing, as some small profit can now go towards funding the Charity.

So, this has been our story so far. We have come a long way, we are still in there expanding and becoming more sophisticated. Now we should examine the success of the programme.

University of Surrey Study 1990 -92

FORESIGHT Audit - 367 couples1990-92

367 COUPLES TOOK PART
327 CONCEIVED (89%)
327 BABIES BORN

NO MISCARRIAGES
NO MALFORMATIONS
NO BIRTH BEFORE 36 WEEKS
NO BABY BELOW 5LB 30Z
NO ADMITTANCE TO SCBU

Comparisons with 327 couples who have birth

	National Average for 327 couples	History of these couples prior pregnancies	FORESIGHT Pregnancy
MISCARRIAGE	92	139	0
STILL BIRTHS	5	11	0
SMALL BABIES (under 51b 8oz)	33	55	1
MALFORMATIONS	11	7	0

FORESIGHT INFERTILE COUPLES

204   FERTILITY PROBLEMS

136   PRIMARY INFERTILITY

68   SECONDARY INFERTILITY

175   BABIES BORN (86%)

     46   COUPLES PREPARED FOR IVF

     30   BABIES BORN (65%)

     158   COUPLES NATURAL CONCEPTION

     145   BABIES BORN (91%)

175   BABIES = 86% OVER ALL

• • • • • • • • • • • • • • • • • •

LOW BIRTH WEIGHT NATIONWIDE

54,000 Low Birth Weight babies, under 5lb 8oz, are born each year in the UK. **(1 in 13 births)**

This has remained **unchanged** in 30 years.

These babies are known to have a greater risk of diabetes and heart disease in later life.

(Michael Crawford & D Barker)

By contrast FORESIGHT babies 1 in 327

In the course of the Study, 1 baby was born weighing 5lb 3oz. The remaining 326 were between 5lb 8oz, and 9lb 3oz.

• • • • • • • • • • • • • • • • • •

MAIN FACTORS IN PARENTAL LIFESTYLES CONTRIBUTING TO LOW BIRTH WEIGHT

1. Poor Nutrition
2. Alcohol & Tobacco
3. The Oral Contraceptive Pill, and other exogenous hormones.
4. Genitourinary Infections
5. Sub-Optimum Mineral Levels
6. High levels of Toxic Metals
7. Over-high Copper Level
8. Allergy & Parasites

The next 7 chapters will take you through a more detailed account of the FORESIGHT Programme for optimum health and optimum sperm production. Our experience has been that, when following this programme, 52.4% of men who formerly suffered from infertility fathered a child. With those men who followed the programme fully we achieved 66.2%. We hope the readers of this book will find that their success rate is even greater!

Where success is not achieved with the FORESIGHT programme alone, we suggest you combine our methods with some additional help as suggested by alternative practitioners in Section II of this book. Sometimes combining more than one approach can produce the solution.

What Can Be Achieved
The FORESIGHT programme has been demonstrated to reduce infertility, miscarriage, malformation, prematurity, small for dates and perinatal death.

Coincidental side effects for the mother include:
Less fatigue and post partum depression.
Less pre-enclamptic toxaemia.
Better lactation, better healing of birth abrasions.
Better maternal instinct - mother-baby bonding.

Coincidental side effects on the baby include:
Good weight and Apgar. *
Better breast-feeding, sleeping, alertness, serenity.
Good general development.
Good cranial/facial structure.
Less crying.
Eczema, colic, diarrhoea, asthma, being extremely rare.

(* Apgar - system of "scoring points" 1 to 10 to assess and record the baby's general condition at birth, invented by a paediatrician called Virginia Apgar.)

Empirical observations with FORESIGHT **School Children indicate:**
Better than average general health, mental acuity, sociability, musicality.

Let us fantasise!

Ultimate World Scene
Healthier Population.
Much Less Disability and/or Chronic Illness.
Better Response to Education.
Happier Marriages/Families/Better Fertility.
Healthier Subsequent Generations!
Gentle Rise, Rather than Fall, in the Collective IQ!
Better Art, Better Music, Better Theatre, Better Architecture!
Less taxpayer's money spent on:

> health-care; including degenerative disease;
> fertility care; care of the handicapped;
> remedial education; delinquency; prisons; crime fighting; war.

One necessary question: *Why do you not find this whole approach on the NHS?*

You may well be wondering (as we are) why more help along the FORESIGHT lines is not available through the normal NHS channels? Except for an excellent service given by the GUI Clinics, (which is not adequately advertised) there is no help, as we understand it, for male infertility.

Sperm donation may be suggested, but this should surely be the very last resort, not the first port of call? Likewise, adoption, particularly as there are almost no babies available for adoption, so this can be a very long and demoralising trail.

The stumbling block appears to lie in the fact that the choice of new policies lies with Government or the Medical Profession, or where the two interface, at the Department of Health. Government representatives have no knowledge of preventative or environmental medicine, so they tend to rely on those who are known as the "expert advisers" (the Humphrey Applebys of Whitehall). The advisers may not have any interest in, or knowledge of, the natural approach to fertility, so their attitude tends to be defensive and dismissive. Much funding of both Government, the Medical Schools and Universities is undertaken by big drug houses, so they, understandably, hold much sway. Their interest lies in promoting the use of the drugs they make. People working in the natural health scene appear less well heeled and therefore, less impressive. They are also not in a position to be so generous, so they tend to be sidelined. Such is the way of the world.

The Medical Profession tends to close ranks and regard an interloper (however economical and successful) as at best, a tedious bore, and at worst, a sinister exploiter! According to the fascinating accounts in Donald Gould's and Jonathan Gascoigne-Hardy's memorable books, students wishing to attend Medical School tend to be selected for their prowess on the rugby field. This seems a curious method of selection for such a sensitive and intellectually demanding profession! However, the willingness to share scrumpox, injury and drunken revelry does produce an insoluble male bonding. Later in life, this solidarity tends to resist all comers, even those bearing good tidings!

One manifestation of this welding together is their unity in their implacable reliance on the "double-blind placebo-controlled crossover trial", in even the most unsuitable circumstances. Any method that has not been tested by this complex but fallible procedure is rejected automatically. The DBPCCO Trial was devised for testing out drugs. The procedure is thus: a randomly selected cohort of patients is divided into two groups. One group receives the drug the medics wish to test, and one a similar looking pill which has no active ingredient. This is known as "the placebo". The bottles of pills are given to different patients to swallow. Neither the patient nor the doctor is allowed to know which bottle contains the active pills. Somewhere along the line, the substances are switched over - also secretly. The patients' progress is noted, and the drug company hopes that while taking the drug, the group will have done better, (and will not have been prone to too many horrendous side effects), while when they were on the placebo they will not have flourished! As you will be able to gather at a glance, this regime could not be applied to a multi-factorial approach, that includes such factors as diet, eschewing tobacco and alcohol, checking the GUI, eliminating allergies and/or parasites, taking supplements, filtering water, etc, etc, etc. It is simply not practicable, even if it was desirable. For obvious reasons, it is also not desirable!

It is therefore impossible for people using the FORESIGHT approach to provide the criteria which would gain us acceptance into the "World of Medicine"!

Natural rude health and reproductive excellence will therefore be forever in the wilderness as far as the medical profession is concerned, (but in very good company, notwithstanding, and in a wilderness with an ever-increasing population!) Gradually the trend will be for people to consult with qualified nutritional therapists, homeopaths and other alternative practitioners who have a more common-sense approach to basic health problems, and who are not inhibited from learning from a simple straightforward presentation of evidence. So, let us look more closely at the alternative ways of tackling male infertility.

CHAPTER 3

NUTRITION AND MENTAL FUNCTION

The Work of Dr Weston Price

We have to start somewhere. Let us start with nutrition. There is fascinating research into the power of good nutrition, starting with Weston Price working in the 1940's, linking nutrition with mental function and reproductive excellence. Dr Price was a dentist in California, who suddenly had the hunch that there must be a cause for dental caries (holes in the teeth). He wondered if it could be diet-related? He pondered this and then he resolved to discover. In the 1930's he and his most enterprising wife donned their solar toupees and set off round the world to examine exactly what all the different races ate, and whether or not their teeth were prone to decay. He wrote the fascinating book, *Nutrition and Physical Degeneration*, detailing his travels and his discoveries, and giving a photographic record of the health and dental development of the people he met.

As he travelled on, he realised that where people were eating their natural diet of fresh, mainly uncooked, foods their normal development was unimpaired. Their teeth were sound. Their skeletal structure was perfect, their muscles were strong. Their sight and hearing were superior to people in more "sophisticated" cultures. They were strong and wise, with a high level of skills and talents, and he saw no retardation among the young, or senility in the old. *Fertility was unimpaired.*

All of this changed, tragically, when Dr Price found the tribes where the "white man's diet" had been introduced.

Refined carbohydrates, cooked and packaged foods had radically changed their society. Illness, tooth decay and reproductive problems plagued the people. Babies were born malformed and retarded. In the fashion of the time it was laconically recorded "the child was an idiot". Malformations were common-place. The people had lost their verve and humour, and the smiles in the photographs were replaced with scowls or miserable expressions. The food had lost its life, and the population had lost their vitality. The calories were devoid of vitamins and minerals, and good health was a thing of the past. These two extreme patterns were evident wherever he travelled among primitive people around the world.

Later, Dr Price came home and conducted research regarding anomalies seen in domestic animals. He found that in all cases where infertility or anomalies in the offspring were present, the fault could be traced back to the deficiency of a crucial nutrient in the animal's diet.

In his book *Nutrition and Physical Degeneration* (published by the Price Pottinger Foundation) we find the following passages:

> *Associated with a fine physical condition the isolated primitive groups have a high level of immunity to many of our modern degenerative processes, including tuberculosis, arthritis, heart disease, and affections of the internal organs. When, however, these individuals have lost this high level of physical excellence a definite lowering in their resistance to the modern degenerative processes has taken place. To illustrate, the narrowing of the facial and dental arch forms of the children of the modernised parents, after they had adopted the white man's food, was accompanied by an increase in susceptibility to pulmonary tuberculosis.*

> *Dr Draper has approached this problem from the data provided in the medical clinics, and therefore, from the characteristics of affected individuals, whereas my approach has been through a study of the primitive groups and the physical changes and disease susceptibilities which occur as a result of their modernisation. The similarity of our conclusions greatly emphasises the importance of the findings of each. Dr Draper has emphasised the importance of the face and of the dental arches in the general matter of susceptibility to disease.*

> *The more we come to view man as a totality, as an organism which functions as a whole and not as a collection of separate elements, the more do all the special branches*

of medicine become fused with the general concept which forms the basis of this discussion, namely, the relation of the human organisation as a whole to those various reactions of maladjustment with environment which we call disease.

If only Dr Price and Dr Draper had been listened to in the 1940's, when all of this was first written, and medicine had taken the path of examining the food and the environment for the sources of illness and degeneration, **what** integrity they would have maintained, and **what** advances mankind could have achieved in the interim.

Instead, we took the wrong turning. Consequently we have been spiralling downwards with the constant intervention of ever more expensive drugs and techniques, produced to mask the symptoms of nutrient deficiencies, allergic illness that is the body's reaction to polluting substances, and ultimately all forms of degenerative disintegration. *No wonder conception is elusive.*

Dr Price goes on to present important data on the vital role played by Vitamin A in the development of the eye which was being investigated in the 1930's by Sherman, who brought to light that fact that "*an amount of Vitamin A sufficient to support normal growth and maintain every appearance of good health in animals, may still be insufficient to meet the added nutritive demands of successful reproduction and lactation.*"

He drew attention to the fact that reproductive problems were often associated with lung disease. In those days pulmonary tuberculosis was the prevalent disease to which younger people were prone when the nutrition, and therefore the immune system, was inadequate. He maintained that an optimum level of Vitamin A was not only necessary for growing children, but for adults as well, "*if a high degree of health and vigour are to be maintained.*"

A further team of investigators, Hart and Gilbert, found that weak or dead calves were born to cattle who were short of Vitamin A. Many of these had eye lesions, or developed eye lesions after birth. They were also prone to "white scours" (pale diarrhoea).

Another researcher called Sure found that lack of Vitamin A produced "*in females a lack of oestrus and ovulation resulting in sterility*", even when the diet contained plenty of Vitamin E.

Another experiment was made by Professor Fred Hale, of Texas, who did a series of experiments mating pigs where the mother was deprived of Vitamin A. Piglets were born without eyes, and suffering paralysis and spasms.

When the sow was given a single dose of cod liver oil before mating, the outcome was somewhat improved, but all piglets were still born blind, although they did have eyes in most cases.

Dr Price went on to describe the work on the paternal side of reproduction:

> *"There are few if any problems connected with modern degeneration on which so much light is thrown as that supplied by recent investigations on the problems of paternal responsibility for defects in the offspring. There are several reasons for this. Because the mother has the sole responsibility for the nourishment of the fetus during the formative period and she alone provides the handicaps incident to the process of birth, it is very natural that defects are practically all interpreted as being associated with these processes. This unfortunately, has been embarrassed further by the fact that since distortions in behaviour do not appear until sometime after birth, normality was largely assumed to be present up to the time of their appearance, and therefore of necessity would be contributions from the child's environment. Hence the entire problem of the role of the sex cells through controlling the architecture of the body including the brain has been largely overlooked. Very important light is thrown on this problem in the data provided on a dachshund pup with cleft palate and a very severe spinal deformity. The highly significant circumstance is the fact that these same deformities not only appeared also in another pup of this same litter but in one pup in each of three other litters about the same time. While four mothers were involved these four litters were all sired by one father. The paternal responsibility is clearly established . . . "*

> In corresponding with Professor Hale, I inquired whether they had information as to the effect of vitamin A deficiency on the sire. He replied, ***"If we reduced the vitamin A content of the body of the sire, he would become sterile and, therefore, we could not try this procedure."*** The question arises as to what the effect would be of a less severe depletion of vitamin A of both parents.

It is a very easy matter to place the full responsibility on the mother, when defects develop in the children. These data indicate that either parent may contribute directly to certain of the defects of the children, due to defects in the germ plasm.

Dr Weston Price saw another very interesting case, when he was on his travels around the world. He met a "full blooded Eskimo woman" who had married, as her second husband, a white man. She made her normal Eskimo diet for herself, but prepared the food he was used to for him. She had a total of 26 children (yes!) but Dr Price found she had no tooth decay. (Tooth decay is one of the first signs of inadequate nutrition). The husband had "*rampant tooth decay and a marked abnormality in the development of the face and of the dental arches*". Several of his daughters had narrow dental arches, one it seems had the typical narrow pelvis seen in Western women, which makes childbirth so difficult. Clearly, good maternal nutritional status alone is **not enough!**

A further study of pigs was done by a researcher called Mackenzie, who mated a sire (boar) known to have defective sperm to two groups of sows. Sows mated with this boar could produce normal piglets when they themselves had access to pasture. When they did not, the rate of deformity was very high. The two groups of sows were enclosed, and again the group without the access to pasture produced large numbers of deformed young.

Dr Price:

> "*This emphasises the need for the vitamins and minerals that are provided in natural foods, particularly vitamin A and seems to relate to the studies of Hale in which the absence of vitamin A produced gross defects. These studies*

on domestic animals strongly emphasise the necessity that both parents shall have adequate nutrition before conception occurs and subsequently for the mother."

Dr Price continues . . .

"Williams states that Loje has observed ten grossly deformed calves of a particular type that were traced to the same sire; also a series of five with this deformity reported by Hutt were traced to one sire. Among the deformities in domestic animals cleft palate or absence of palate is very common. These studies on domestic animals strongly emphasise two facts; first, that deformities among these animals are very similar to those that develop in humans, and second, that the defects are largely related to the original germ cells and that the male may provide the defect quite as well as the female . . . "

Also, from the same book as above, Dr Price conducted an interesting study with human semen.

"Moench and Holt of the Cornell Medical School and New York hospital have made important studies on humans and have found a very high incidence of sterility when abnormal forms of spermatozoa reached 25%. Among the abnormal forms they found one particular family with a particular type of abnormal sperm reaching 12%. Their breeding record was decidedly bad, and fetal malformations repeatedly occurred. In their group, in 63 sterile matings the men were normal 21 times and abnormal 37 times. They listed over 40 different abnormal or deformed types of sperm. They conclude:

1. *In normal semen the abnormal sperm heads do not exceed 19 to 20%.*

2. *When the sperm head abnormalities reach 20 to 23%, impaired fertility can be assumed.*

3. *When the sperm head abnormalities are above 25%, clinical sterility is usually present."*

It is interesting that these comments were made in the 1940's. Today we accept abnormalities at this level and well above this level as inevitable. We should all become more aware. Not just that there is a planetary problem, but also of what we can do about it in our own backyard.

Dr Price then goes on to describe work done by 2 German surgeons who were involved in enforcing the sterilisation law in Berlin at this time. I think we should take what good we can from this vile situation, as we do from the animal studies. At least all the sacrifices made will not have been entirely in vain, if they contribute to a positive knowledge pool, and are used henceforth for good purposes.

It was thought at that time that a normal man would produce up to 19% defective sperm. It was found the chronic alcoholic patient produced 75% defective. The mentally defective male produced 62% defective, those suffering from hereditary deafness 62% defective, and those suffering hereditary blindness 75%. (This latter group may have been Vitamin A deficient from birth). Those suffering epilepsy and schizophrenia 54 - 58% defective.

There would be connections with prenatal nutrient deficiency especially vitamin deficiencies, and zinc, selenium and manganese, with all of the above groups.

In a personal communication to Dr Price, Professor TS Sutton of the College of Agriculture, Ohio State University, makes the following observation:

> *"For several years we have been interested in the study of the effects of vitamin A deficiency. Right now our main consideration is the effect of this deficiency on reproduction. We find that a diet low in vitamin A will cause reproductive failure, which seems to be caused chiefly by a degeneration of the germinal epithelium of the gonad. This is particularly true in the case of the male. I think we have rather convincing evidence that this is a direct dietary damage to the gonad (ovary or testis), rather than a disruption of the endocrine balance which might result in sterility as appears to be the case in vitamin B deficiency."*

The degenerative processes which occur in nerve tissues due to vitamin A deficiency have been studied by Professor Sutton and his associates. They have been able to show detailed progressive degeneration within nerve fibres as a result of vitamin A deficiency.

In the light of the newer information it is quite clear why we may have any one of the following distinct expressions in the reproductive process, namely, physical excellence of succeeding generations (such as obtains among many of the primitive races as I have shown); complete reproductive failure or sterility or partial failure resulting in defectives of various types at the borderline between these two phases. It is the rapid and progressive increase in this last group which constitutes the progressive degeneration of our modern civilisation.

One of the main problems in this study has to do with the relation of nutrition to the modification of the growth of the child, both in its formative period and in the stage of adolescence. I have shown that in many of these primitive racial stocks there occurs in the first generation after the displacement of native foods by imported foods a marked change in facial and dental arch forms. These changes happen most frequently in the later children in the families and come about notwithstanding the impact of heredity through all the previous generations of excellent physical development. Clinically, the evidence is abundant, that this change occurs in these primitive racial stocks regardless of colour, geographic location, temperature, and climate. We are apparently dealing here with a factor which, while it may be related to the germ plasm and to the prenatal growth period, clearly involves other forces than those that are at work in the case of hereditary defectives. Since these changes have to do directly with disturbances in growth of the head, particularly of the face and of the dental arches, we are concerned with such evidence as may be available as to the nature of the forces that readily affect the anatomy of the skull.

The general architecture of the body is apparently determined primarily by the health of the two germ cells at the time of their union. This architectural design may not be completely fulfilled due to interference with nutritive processes both before and after birth. In this large problem of the relationship between physical design of the body and resistance or susceptibility to disease, we may have determining factors operating at different periods in prenatal and postnatal growth. The accumulating evidence strongly emphasises that disease susceptibility is a widely variable factor and associated with certain types of developmental disturbances. "

If only more attention had been paid to all this work in the 1950's! How much suffering could have been saved!

• • • • • • • • • • • • • • • • • • •

The Recent FORESIGHT Leaflet on Vitamin A
Vitamin A in Pregnancy

The measurement of Vitamin A has recently been changed from the old "iu" (international units), with which we were all familiar, to the new "European Correctness" of "mcg" or micro-grams.

These two measurements do not reflect exactly the same thing.

The international units used to give the potency of the source (which can vary with the oil soluble vitamins). The mcg only gives the weight. However, the powers-that-be have ruled that to convert iu of Vitamin A to mcg, we divide by 3.33, and so for all practical purposes this will now have to serve us. To avoid confusion we will give both measurements in this leaflet, as you may find either in papers, or on tubs of supplements.

For pregnancy, FORESIGHT advises 2,500iu (833mcg) - 5,000iu (1,501mcg).

Vitamin A excess can be dangerous in pregnancy, but so can Vitamin A deficiency. The dangers of Vitamin A deficiency have been too little understood or published over the last decade.

Scientific advice on what constitutes excess Vitamin A is very variable. The Denner Report quoted 10,000iu (3,003mcg). Professor Merlyn Werbach of the University of California (arguably the world authority on fetal nutrition) says 40,000iu (12,012mcg). An Australian source gives 25,000iu (7,507mcg). FORESIGHT programmes are always very conservative, as the obvious approach is to give enough to avoid any danger of deficiency, while giving very little more than this, to be sure of staying within the safe limit.

The maximum we usually give is:

2 x FORESIGHT Vitamin Supplements	=	2,500iu (750mcg) plus
4 x Selenium ACE	=	1,732iu (520mcg)
Total Given	=	4,232iu (1,270mcg)

The minimum we give is the 2,500iu (750mcg) present in two FORESIGHT Vitamins.

Even our most generous programmes give less than half the most conservative upper limit, which was the Denner Report's 10,000iu (3,003mcg).

It is interesting to note in this context that during the war (when, despite rationing, most people's diet was more nutritious than that of today), the Government decreed all pregnant women should have "a teaspoonful of cod liver oil" daily. It is hard to assess the amount of Vitamin A, as a lot would have depended on the size of the teaspoon, but it is likely to have been in the region of 5,000iu (1,501mcg). At the present time, in the USA, pregnant women are given 5,000iu (1,501mcg) Vitamin A daily. In some areas of Australia, they are given 10,000iu (3,003mcg). UNESCO campaigns for funding to give Vitamin A to pregnant mothers in the Third World to stop babies from being born blind.

In 24 years of running FORESIGHT we have not seen any of the deformities listed above in "our" babies. I would not therefore be tempted to supplement above 5,000iu (1,501mcg), although you could probably take up to 10,000iu (3,003mcg) without harm.

However, I think there could be a case made out for a little more with the multiple births, especially triplets.

I would also not be confused or bullied into taking less than 2,500iu (750mcg) as this could lead to the risk of serious malformations. 45,000 babies (1 baby in 16) are now born in Britain with malformations annually. The largest groups include those with malformations listed above which are proven by scientific research to be due to Vitamin A deficiency. This is a tragedy probably greater than the thalidomide debacle, and it should be more easily preventable, as all the research is out there, and has been for many years.

At the present time, The Department of Health (DoH), say they "*have no position on Vitamin A in pregnancy*". They passed me on to the Food Standards Agency who passed me back to the DoH. On second contact, we have had an exchange of correspondence that you will find on our website.

We continue to advise women to take between 2,500iu (750mcg) and 4,232iu (1,270mcg) daily, before and throughout pregnancy.

You are welcome to take this leaflet to your GP, midwife or health visitor if this would be helpful. If they (or you) have any scientific papers that contradicts what I am saying, or supports it, I would be particularly grateful to be sent copies of these, as I would be very interested to study them.

• • • • • • • • • • • • • • • • • • •

Another stalwart pioneer of Dr Price's era was Dr Frank Pottinger. Work by Dr Pottinger, with cats, had proved how allergies and other illnesses of the immune system could be brought into being, or eliminated, in succeeding generations, by the way the cats were fed.

Dr Pottinger had two runs, with cats and their kittens kept in each.

One group was fed raw meat and raw (unpasteurised) milk, while those in the second run were fed cooked meat and pasteurised milk.

The cats on the raw diet produced fine healthy kittens with no problems. The cats on the cooked and pasteurised food produced sickly kittens with runny eyes and noses, wheezy chests and poor coats. (Analagous to all the common problems we talk about today as "allergies" in the children!)

Significantly, when the trial was over and the cats were re-homed, the potency of their excreta was revealed. The weeds that grew in the first run were healthier and more prolific than those in the second. Dr Pottinger planted beans in both runs. The bean plants in the first run produced beans well in excess of those produced in the second. By such simple experiments, profound truths were revealed. **Whole foods mean superior reproduction for both animal and plant life.**

The Work of Dr Carl Pfeiffer and Other Researchers

Some quarter of a century later, another dogged pioneer, and a man of huge charm, was *Dr Carl Pfeiffer*, of New Jersey. For over 30 years he was studying the effects of trace minerals on brain development and brain function, and also on sexual function, working with people with schizophrenia. **Like Dr Weston Price, he found that growth, mental development, sexual function and fertility were all extremely dependant on the levels of trace minerals and vitamins in the diet.**

He made huge advances with the treatment of degenerative disease and mental illness by measuring and correcting trace mineral deficiencies. He was able to combat sexual dysfunction in male patients using vitamins, zinc, manganese, calcium, magnesium and other nutrients.

His work was supported by that of *Dr Ananda Prasad,* in Egypt, who was doing a lot of work with boys who suffered from dwarfism, mental impairment, under-development of their sexual organs and many chronic illnesses due to lack of zinc. The Egyptian soil lacked zinc, and so throughout the region, the food was inadequate in this respect, and these problems were rife.

Later, the work of *Doctors Oberleas and Caldwell,* at Wayne State University, included studying the deterioration in mental function of rats and mice when they were deprived of zinc, iron, magnesium and manganese. Young rats are usually well able to cope with complex mazes, respond in time to electronic warnings of painful shocks, etc. The deprived rats were fazed and panicked by such simple tasks, while those who had not been deprived took them in their stride.

In Miami, *Doctors Riopele and Hubbard,* researched with mice and rats, and linked their central nervous system deterioration with manganese deficiency. It was found that when they were deprived of manganese before birth, the young rats could not right themselves when placed on their backs. This may have been due to underdevelopment of the otiliths in the middle ear. Their righting reflexes and their ability to balance were chronically impaired by lack of prenatal manganese.

Professor EJ Underwood, in Australia, undertook studies of all the trace minerals and how deficiencies affected reproductive performance. Low zinc, selenium and manganese in particular were found to cause infertility. Also, these deficiencies caused malformations in children and in the young of small research animals such as rats, rabbits and mice, and in those of domestic livestock, such as cows and sheep.

They were all mentally impaired or physically damaged by the lack of certain trace minerals in their diet. *Fertility in particular was found to be destroyed by a shortage of zinc, and/or manganese, and/or selenium..*

Professor Saner, and colleagues in the USA, studied the young of human mothers who had been manganese deficient during pregnancy, and found spina bifida, hydrocephalus and other gross deformities of the central nervous system in these babies.

Professor Lucille Hurley, working in California University with rats and mice, found spina bifida and other major malformations in the young of those who were kept short of zinc and/or manganese prior to conception.

Professor Bert Vallee, at Harvard University Medical School working with a large number of experimental animals of different species, found premature birth was the direct result of copper/zinc imbalance, (ie: high copper and low zinc), in the mother. In the last trimester of pregnancy the copper rises in the blood, while the zinc is all packed into the placenta. Thus the ratio of copper (a brain stimulant) over the level of zinc is raised in the brain. This starts the phenomenon of birth. If the blood has extra copper and low zinc early on in the pregnancy, and this is not corrected at this stage, this can cause premature birth and miscarriage.

After birth, most animals eat the placenta. Professor Vallee found that this restored the copper/zinc balance within 96 hours of birth. Women who do not have zinc supplementation after birth may become hyperstimulated and depressed due to the continual high copper level in the brain.

Dr Pfeiffer found high copper/low zinc in schizophrenic patients, it is also seen in hyperactive and allergic children. Copper water pipes causing high copper levels in domestic water supplies may compound these problems in some areas.

Dr Isobel Jennings, veterinary pathologist of Cambridge University did a massive amount of work with a number of different species and reported how reproduction was badly affected by a lack of vitamins.

All the major deformities that are constantly seen in handicapped children were seen in experimental animals, as a result of deficiencies of Vitamins A, D, E and many of the B-complex vitamins. In her book Vitamins in Endocrine Metabolism, (William Heinemann Medical Press, 1972), she puts it so well:

> *"Hormonal and vitamin imbalances which cause malaise or even pass unnoticed in post-natal life, may have a disastrous effect on the developing fetus. The rapid rate of growth of embryonic cells, which far surpasses that of most tumour cells, is the basic factor which determines the exaggerated fetal response to injurious stimuli. Interference with growth or metabolism of developing cells at an early stage is reflected ultimately in alterations at the stage of differentiation, with resulting malformations or impaired function of developing organs and tissues. The embryonic cell has much in common with the malignant cell, including high mitotic rate, and lack of differentiation in the early stages.*
>
> *Early fetal development depends to a certain extent on hormones supplied by the maternal endocrine organs and the placenta and on vitamins and other food factors derived from the maternal blood supply. Eventually, however, each fetal endocrine organ grows, differentiates and matures, and in those animals which are born at a relatively well developed state, produce their own hormones, many of which are essential for further normal development of their receptor organs and tissues. As each organ develops, it influences the growth and maturation of other organs, and eventually the functional relationships between endocrine glands characteristic of post-natal life become established.*
>
> *Many of the experimentally induced vitamin deficiencies cause malformations identical with those reputed to be hereditary in origin. As a rule, the demands of the mother for vitamins take priority over fetal demands, so that in many cases there may be no sign of maternal deficiency*

in essential food factors, while at the same time the fetus may be suffering marked deficiency. This means that a marginal maternal deficiency, which is very difficult to detect, may have grave consequences for the fetus."

All of these studies showed clearly that nutrient deficiency of the ovary and testicle and of the embryo once conception has taken place, do *tragically disadvantage* the subsequent young. Not enough nutrients before conception both in the sperm and in the ova mean imperfectly formed cells in the offspring, this is later reflected as deformity or impaired mental function. The responsibility rests with both the male and the female, and there is a wide spectrum of disadvantage. If there is only a small level of deficiency in one or other parent, the baby may be small or may be malformed. If the deficiency becomes more marked, the young are born earlier and earlier, until the curtailed gestation period is incompatible with life. The spontaneous abortions take place earlier and earlier, then, when the deficiencies are sufficiently severe, implantation and/or conception will not take place at all.

It would seem feasible inducing infertility during periods of nutritional deficiency may be part of a primitive Grand Plan of Nature. If there is not enough food to go around, then many fewer mouths to be fed will be an advantage. *"Until better times"* says Nature, *"let's close down the baby factories!"*

Both the ova and the sperm need to be fully nourished to be able to spring forth new life. We are all of us part of a continuum of life that started we know not where. Whether we sprang from Adam and Eve and their exceptionally difficult offspring, or from some admirably enterprising little amoeba, or whether we came from some other planet, we know not where or when, as the Red Indians maintain, it matters not. We have been going a very long time. We know enough to make a fist of working towards a Better Planet for One and All. So don't lets have it all end here, just for want of a bit more effort and organisation on our part!

INFORMATION FROM SOME RESEARCH PAPERS ON SPECIFIC NUTRIENTS

The following research is compiled from the work of Dr Weston Price, Dr Frank Pottinger, Dr Roger Williams, Adelle Davies, Dr Carl Pfeiffer, Dr EJ Underwood of Australia, and others. The disadvantages listed as Maternal Deficiency will, in almost every case, apply equally to the adult male. To read through the lists will help to identify the source of many health problems.

Trace Elements and Preconceptual Care

CALCIUM

- Maternal deficiency
  * Allergy, tooth decay, back pain, osteoporosis, insomnia, irritability, nervousness, uneven heartbeat, indigestion, stomach cramps and spasms, constipation, pre-menstrual tension and cramping of the uterus.

- Foetal deficiency
  * Rickets and later tooth decay. High raised palate.

MAGNESIUM

- Maternal deficiency
  * Allergy, impaired protein synthesis, enzyme deficiencies, tremor, twitching and convulsions, panic attacks, insomnia, uneven heartbeat, leg and foot cramps, pre-menstrual tension, period pains, depression, poor memory, confusion, disorientation, hyperactivity, irritability, anxiety, nightmares, and increased sensitivity to noise. Stones may form in the kidneys.

- Foetal deficiency
  * Congenital abnormalities, calcium deposits and other abnormalities of the heart cells, anorexia, convulsions and perinatal death.

POTASSIUM

- Maternal deficiency
  * Acid urine, nervous irritability, disorientation, fatigue, listlessness, insomnia, muscle weakness, uneven heartbeat, constipation, cramping muscles, low blood sugar and coma.

- Foetal deficiency
  * Possible low blood sugar, and/or constipation in the new born.

IRON

- Maternal deficiency
  * Anaemia, weakness, shortage of breath, excessive fatigue, depression, confusion, poor memory and poor resistance to infection.

- Foetal deficiency
  * Eye defects, bone defects, brain defects and neonatal mortality.

  * Iron deficiency is rare however

  * Iron excess can be toxic. Excessive supplementation can cause constipation and vomiting and can lead to miscarriage.

  * Recent work from Germany has linked excessive iron supplementation to neonatal jaundice.

CHROMIUM

- Maternal deficiency
  * Poor sugar handling, arteriosclerosis, hypertension and diabetes. Sugar and alcohol consumption reduces chromium.

- Foetal deficiency
  * Eye abnormalities.

  * Possible link with later development of diabetes.

COBALT

- Maternal deficiency
  - * Vitamin B12 deficiency, can give pernicious anaemia. Vitamin B12 deficiency may be present in vegetarians and vegans, in people taking cleansing programmes with high doses of Vitamin C or eating a diet high in refined carbohydrates and/or alcohol.

- Foetal deficiency
  - * Problems are not recorded. The fetus has quite efficient mechanisms for storing Vitamin B 12.

COPPER

- Maternal deficiency
  - * Porous bones, loss of hair, demyelination and anaemia.

- Foetal deficiency
  - * Depressed growth rate, de-pigmentation, anaemia, fine fragile bones, ataxia, small brain, perinatal mortality.

  - * Copper deficiency is very rare however

  - * Copper excess is much more common, resulting, in women, from the contraceptive pill or the fertility drugs. This can result in zinc and manganese deficiency with the resulting miscarriages, premature births, malformations and retardation.

MANGANESE

- Maternal deficiency
  - * Enzyme deficiencies (allergy), poor fat metabolism, epilepsy, thought confusion, poor memory, poor thyroid function, depression.

  - * NB - After the birth, manganese deficiency can lead to hormonal deficiencies resulting in postpartum depression and lack of bonding, which can cause rejection of the baby.

- Foetal deficiency
  * Malformation of the inner ear, ataxia, bone malformation, lack of co-ordination, head retraction, tremor, lack of righting reflexes, hyperactivity, hyper-irritability, faulty cartilage and bone matrix formation, heart problems, epilepsy, convulsions, learning difficulties, allergy, muscle weakness.

NICKEL

- Maternal deficiency
  * Cirrhosis of the liver and chronic kidney failure.

- Foetal deficiency
  * Heart defects, kidney defects, liver defects, neonatal death.

  * Excess of nickel can also be toxic, but this has never been seen in FORESIGHT testing. Occasionally, nickel is low in people with urinary tract infections.

SELENIUM

- Maternal deficiency
  * Muscle weakness, muscular dystrophy, swelling, internal haemorrhages, atrophy of the pancreas, liver necrosis, cataract, cancer, allergy to inhaled substances (eg dust mite, pollen, dandruff), asthma.

  * American research has linked selenium deficiency with chromosome damage, including Down's Syndrome. FORESIGHT research appears to confirm this.

  * Selenium will combine with toxic metals and help to cleanse these from the body. We use this in combination with Vitamin C and garlic.

  * It is interesting to note that fluoride is antagonistic to selenium. Studies in America have found a fourfold increase in Down's Syndrome births where the water has been fluoridated.

* Excessive supplementation of selenium however can be toxic.
* Selenium-containing shampoos should be avoided prior to and during pregnancy.

- Foetal deficiency
  * Stillbirth, growth retardation, testicular damage, poor muscle tone, an increase in the incidence of Down's Syndrome has been recorded and weakness of the lungs.

ZINC

- Maternal deficiency
  * Poor maintenance of bones, muscles, eyes, organs, teeth. Poor liver function and carotene conversion. White spots on nails, stretch marks, lank hair, acne, painful knee and hip joints, cold extremities, lack of taste and smell, anorexia, body and breath odour.

    In women, lack of menstruation and ovulation (thus infertility). Where conception does take place, miscarriage or premature birth, insomnia and extreme fatigue. Extended parturition (labour fade).

  * After birth: fatigue, postpartum depression, rejection of infant, lactation failure, poor wound healing, and increased susceptibility to infections.

- Foetal deficiency
  * Growth retardation, anorexia, colic, diarrhoea, apathy, lethargy, seborrhoea, loss of hair, defects in eyes, kidneys, brain and bones (skeletal malformations). Spina Bifida, cleft palate, heart defects. Faulty trunk and limb development, curvature of the spine, reduced brain size, heart problems and small eyes. *Also undescended testicles or no testicles in the male.*

  * Later this can manifest as allergic illness, eczema, learning difficulties and hyperactivity. Growth retardation, especially in the male.

IODINE

- Maternal deficiency
    * Fatigue, lethargy, increased susceptibility to cold, low libido, anorexia, slow pulse, low blood pressure, rapid weight gain, high blood cholesterol, heart disease and cancer.

- Foetal deficiency
    * Growth and mental development are retarded.

VANADIUM

- Maternal deficiency
    * Infertility and possibly depression.

- Foetal deficiency
    * Small birth weight and increased perinatal death.

TOXIC METALS - LEAD AND CADMIUM EXCESS

- Maternal excess
    * Headaches, diarrhoea, fatigue, increased risk of cancer.

- Foetal excess
    * Stillbirth, perinatal death, impaired weight gain.

    * Later children exhibit significantly impaired IQ, non-adaptive classroom behaviour, neuropsychological deficits, less favourable development through the first year of life.

    * Cadmium has a strong negative effect on verbal IQ, and lead a stronger negative effect upon IQ.

    * Later children exhibit many so-called "minor health problems" - such as allergic syndromes, eczema, epilepsy, hyperactivity, dyslexia. (These are not "minor" to the family or the child!)

From "Vitamins in Endocrine Metabolism" by Isobel Jennings, MRCVS, Cambridge (1972)

As well as this work on minerals - from American and Australian sources - we have the following information on vitamins from our own Isabel Jennings, the veterinary biochemist and pathologist mentioned in the last chapter. This is work from her animal studies.

Foetal animal studies by a veterinary pathologist

Vitamin A

Excess	Deficiency
Cranial anomalies	No eyes
Cleft Palate	Micropthalmas (small eyes, possibly impaired sight)
Hare Lip	Blindness
Eye defects	Hydrocephalus (water on the brain)
Hydrocephalus	Cardiovascular Anomalies
Spina Bifida	Urogenital Anomalies
Exencephalus (malformed brain & skull)	Diaphragmatic Hernia
	Hypospadia (deformed penis)
	Cryptorchidism (undescended testicles)

B Complex Vitamins

Figures given in brackets before the vitamin indicate the percentage of vitamin left in refined (white) flour

(23%) Vitamin B1 (Thiamine) Deficiency

Sterility or relative infertility
Undersized young
High perinatal mortality
Poor "maze learning" ability

(20%) Vitamin B2 (Riboflavin) Deficiency
Sterility. Stillbirth
"Small, misshapen fetuses"
Reduced oxygen consumption in liver
Reduced enzyme activity
Blood disorders
Micromelia (short little finger)
Short mandibles (poorly formed jaws)
Cleft Palate
Syndactilism (joined fingers & toes)
Oedema and anaemia
Degeneration of Wolffian bodies (impaired kidney development)

(19%) Vitamin B3 (Nicotinamide) Deficiency
Cleft Lip and Palate
Hind Limb Defects

(50%) Vitamin B5 (Pantothenate) Deficiency
Interventrical Septal Defects (heart malformation)
Anomalies of the Aortic Arch (heart malformation)
Cleft Palate
Club Foot
Hydronephrosis (problems with kidneys and urinary system)
Hydroureter (problems with kidneys and urinary system)
Ectopic Gonads (misplaced glands)
Foetal Death/Resorption
Undersized Young
Lack of Myelination
Anomalies of the Nervous System

(33%) Folate Deficiency
Foetal Death/Resorption
Cleft Palate
Hare Lip
Malformation of the:
        Limbs/Heart/Diaphragm/Skeletal System/
        Blood Vessels/Adrenals and/or Eyes
Spina Bifida

Kidney and Lung Underdevelopment
Cataracts
Brain Deformities
Oedema and Anaemia

Biotin Deficiency
Foetal Death/Resorption
Perinatal Death
Degenerative Changes in Heart, Blood Vessels and Liver

Vitamin D Deficiency
Skeletal Deformities
Skull Deformity
High Raised Palate

(14%) Vitamin E Deficiency
Sterility
Foetal Death/Resorption
Exencephally
Hydrocephalus
Syndactyly
Oedema

Essential Fatty Acid Deficiency
Failure to Maintain Growth
Degenerative Changes in Blood Vessels
Perinatal Death
Poor Performance in "Maze Tests".

We have mentioned in the previous pages (not to say plundered at some length) the work of Dr Weston Price. He travelled the world in many cases to meet so-called primitive peoples, with the originally quite modest ambition of wishing to find why some people had dental caries and others did not. As with FORESIGHT, he expanded his remit as his knowledge grew! As the years went by, he realised that those who had no dental caries also had no orthodontal problems. If the teeth were properly made, the jaw and palate were also perfectly formed. Where there were no orthodontal problems or tooth decay, the skull was perfectly formed and symmetrical. There were no blocked Eustachian tubes or sinuses. The hearing and eyesight were exceptionally good. The intelligence was superior.

Where the skull and brain were perfectly formed and fully functional, the body was also well developed and athletic. The beautiful facial structures, physiques and personalities are shown in the pictures in his unique book *Nutrition & Physical Degeneration* (1940).

Where the "white man's diet" of refined carbohydrates and sugar had reached the trading post and had replaced the natural diet of fresh raw, unrefined foods, within one generation the deterioration was obvious. The pictures demonstrate this very clearly. The book compares and contrasts the faces of those on a natural healthy diet, and those on the poor substitutes that most of us are eating (at least some of the time) today! *As the general health deteriorated, so did the fertility.*

Dr Price also worked as the dental officer to a young person's penitentiary and again demonstrated the link between these deprived youngsters' inadequate diet, their decaying teeth, poorly formed palates - high raised palates - their cramped skull development and their inadequate mental development. This had led them from poor school performance to truancy, and from truancy to a life of crime.

His wonderful book, *Nutrition and Physical Degeneration*, still being published from the Price-Pottinger Foundation in La Mesa, California, should be read by every health professional and every prospective parent prior to conception. *They would never be the same again!*

This work has demonstrated both the link between the lack of nutrients in the womb and the high raised palate, and has also demonstrated the link between the high raised palate, cramped skull development and brain damage.

In this context, it is interesting that in England, Dr June Sharpe, of Godalming, Surrey, (one more pioneering spirit!) did a small survey of palate height, and mental development, in her local schools, that confirmed this work.

A Small Study of Palate Height
conducted by Dr June Sharpe of Godalming, Surrey, UK, in the 1970s.

Palate Height - Normal Primary School - 95 Children Seen

Palate Height	Percentage
Normal	73%
Marginal	9%
High	18%

The percentage of children in normal schooling with dyslexia and other learning difficulties is said to be 20%. The list was given to Dr Sharpe after the examination was completed, and she found that those with problems fell into the Marginal and High Group.

• • • • • • • • • • • • • • • • • • •

Palate Height - School for Children with Learning Difficulties
95 Children Seen

Palate Height	Percentage
Normal	31%
Marginal	5%
High	64%

Note that nearly two out of three come under 'high'!

• • • • • • • • • • • • • • • • • • •

She then visited a home for the Mentally Sub-Normal. They were only able to examine 13 children. Some of the children might have been too emotionally disturbed and/or might have bitten the examiners!

Palate Height - Home for Mentally Subnormal Children
13 Children Seen

Palate Height	Percentage
Normal	15%
Marginal	15%
High	70%

I think this breaks down to only 2 of the retarded children seen had a normally developed palate!

Two more fascinating studies of the effect of nutrients on the development of the unborn:

Lawrence Study

A study was done with a group of mothers who had previously had a spina bifida baby, in South Wales in 1980, by Professor KN Lawrence et al, and published in the British Medical Journal.

174 women who had previously given birth to an infant with spina bifida were recruited and were followed up through their subsequent 186 pregnancies. They were divided up as to those on a "Good Diet", those on a "Fair Diet" and those on a "Poor Diet". Outcomes were as follows:

	Good Diet (no 53)	Fair Diet (no 88)	Poor Diet (no 45)
Miscarriages	0	3	15
Spina Bifida (terminated)	0	0	8

Of those on a "Good" or "Fair" diet, only 3 babies were miscarried out of 141 - making 1 pregnancy in 47. This compares well with the UK average of 1 in 4. Of those on the "Poor" diet, 23 out of 45, or just over half the babies were lost, or were malformed and subsequently terminated.

Canadian Study

This is the Birth Record of a poor mother in Montreal. The birth outcomes were recorded before and after a nutritional programme provided by the Alice Higgins Foundation. This consisted of dietary advice, and the provision of a pint of milk, an egg and an orange per day. Of the first eight children she gave birth to, before dietary advice and food allowances were given, 6 were below 2,500 gms, none were above 2,750 gms, two below 1,750 gms and one of these died. All eight were neurologically damaged and the seven survivors had to be institutionalised.

After the Alice Higgins programme, however, the next 3 births were much happier. The weights ranged between 3,500 gms, and 3,750 gms, and all three children were mentally sound.

**Table 3   Nutritional Supplementation Programme
(Montreal)**

Birthweight record of one mother before and during the Alice Higgins
programme

Cost:
With   - $125 / child
Without   - $3M so far

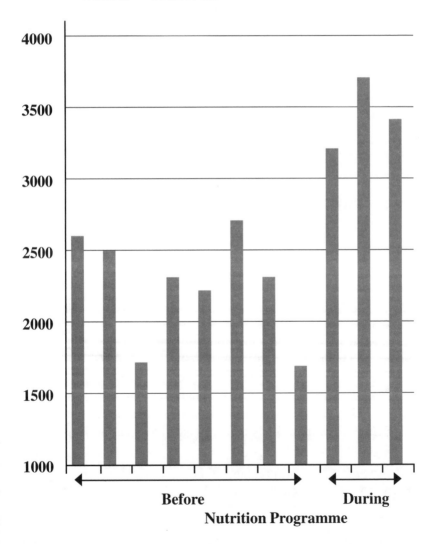

The extra foods provided cost $125 per child. Up to the 1980s, the institutionalising of the seven surviving handicapped children had cost the State $300,000 - and counting.

This is an extreme case, but it is not entirely atypical of what is going on daily in the UK. So many children are being born subtly or overtly handicapped and the family grief is total, the disadvantages can be lifelong, and the tax-payer's impoverishment is spread over lifetimes, and counting.

This is likely to escalate unless we all, every Man Jack of us, make a concerted effort to take things in hand. Research has served to convince us of the vital role played by adequate food in promoting health in pregnancy. We recommend the following books to those wishing to study the background work:

Nutrition & Physical Degeneration - by Dr Weston Price

Nutrition & Health - by Sir Robert McCarrison

Vitamins in Endocrine Metabolism - by Isobel Jennings
(*now out of print, but* FORESIGHT *has off-prints of the chapter on reproduction*)

Nutrition Against Disease - by Dr Roger Williams

Diet & Disease - by Cheraskin, Ringsdorf and Clark

What We Eat Today - by Professor Michael Crawford

More topically the NACNE Report has criticised the level of animal fat, sugar and other refined carbohydrates in the UK diet. In stressing the importance of whole grains, vegetables and fruit, NACNE goes a long way towards the type of diet we would recommend to provide the vitamins, minerals and essential fatty acids needed for a successful pregnancy.

In fact all authoritative writers on diet in recent years have stressed that far too much sugar has been consumed in the Western World. Much is used in combination with nutrient depleted refined flour, which would otherwise have little flavour.

Table 4

Dr Henry Schroeder, Battleborough, Vermont

REFINED FLOUR CONTAINS:

(when compared with amounts
found in wholewheat flour, taken as 100%)

Thiamine	23%	Chromium	13%
Riboflavin	20%	Manganese	9%
Nicotinamide	19%	Iron	19%
Pyridoxine	29%	Cobalt	13%
Pantothenate	50%	Copper	10-30%
Folic Acid	33%	Zinc	17%
Vitamin E	14%	Molybdenum	50%
Magnesium	17%		

No wonder white flour does not do a lot for us! This goes for all the white flour products products on the shelves of the supermarkets: bread, cakes, biscuits, sponge puddings, pizza, pasta, things in sauces, soups, things in batter, breadcrumbs and pastry . . .

All providing about one-fifth of the nutrients that should be contained in them.

UK Sugar Consumption

- In the 19th Century, average sugar consumption was **8lbs** per year, per person - recipes recommended "a pinch"

- In the 20th Century, the consumption has risen to **90lbs** per year, per person. Over **11** times the quantity!

According to Dr Elizabeth Lodge Rees of California the incidence of diabetes in USA has risen steadily in ratio with the amount of sugar purchased in the States. White sugar is particularly damaging as vitamins of the B-complex and trace minerals such as zinc, manganese, chromium, selenium and cobalt are all removed by the refining process. As these substances are necessary for the body to effect the metabolism of sugar, so the white sugar squanders these nutrients from the body's reserves.

Many authoritative writers, such as the late *Professor Carl Pfeiffer* of New Jersey, the late *Dr David Horrobin* of Montreal, *Dr Donald Oberleas* of Kentucky, the late *Isobel Jennings* of Cambridge, *Professor Lucille Hurley* of California and *Professor Bert Vallee* of Harvard University have drawn attention to the connection between lack of these nutrients and mental illness, retarded mental and physical development in the human population and also reproductive disasters in experimental animals. Also the work of the late *Dr Ben Feingold* of California stressed the dangers to small children of food additives such as artificial flavours, colourings and preservatives. Working with hyperactive children over many years, Dr Feingold believed that many of these chemicals were at least a contributory cause of hyperactivity and learning difficulties in children. In other words that they caused temporary or permanent brain malfunction.

Research which followed found that, in all but 15% of children studied, there were other additional causes such as food allergies, heavy metal(s) contamination or specific deficiencies. However the Hyperactive Children's Support Group in this country have found that many thousands of hyperactive children have been considerably helped by a wholefood diet free from chemical additives. Prof Soothill of Great Ormond St Hospital for Sick Children has published a paper outlining the improvement in the incidence of childhood migraine or in hyperactivity following dietary manipulation. It would seem to follow that as these additives can affect the brain of a school-age child, their effect on the brain of a newborn baby may be even more devastating.

To help parents sort their way through the Supermarket jungle, FORESIGHT has prepared a booklet, 'Find Out', giving the number and name of each additive and the effect it can have on the body. We have emphasised that those deemed unsuitable for small children should also be avoided by the pregnant and nursing mother and the prospective father - and that means preconceptually too by those who are planning a pregnancy.

So now let us look at the advice written for FORESIGHT Members by *Louise Templeton, BDA*.

THE WHOLEFOOD DIET

Golden Rules

Bread and Cereals (Organic)

For those who are not sensitive to wheat, organic whole-wheat bread containing 100% of the grain is a good energy food. Organically grown whole-wheat flour is available with the Soil Association Label. This guarantees that it is produced without the use of artificial fertilisers, insecticide or fungicide sprays. Whole-wheat bread, scones, cakes, biscuits etc can be made with this flour.

100% organic whole-grain breakfast cereals are available. Dove Farm, Whole Earth, Nature's Path, and some own brands are now widely available in the Supermarkets, and hopefully more organic whole-grain cereals will appear, watch the spaces!

There are muesli/fruit/seed and nut bars for snacks. A high fibre porridge can be made from oatflakes, oatmeal, millet, pot barley, polenta (corn) or brown rice flakes.

There are varieties of organic whole-grain hard bread on the market, and different types of organic whole-wheat biscuit can be bought, especially HRH's Duchy Originals. Sweet biscuits can be made at home using raw sugar, honey or molasses and organic whole-wheat flour - also flapjacks with oatflakes or oatmeal.

Jams and marmalade made without artificial flavouring and colouring and sweetened with unrefined sugar, honey, apple juice etc, are now available - or can be made at home.

Gluten-free, Wheat-free (for those who cannot tolerate gluten)
Rice, corn, potato, soya, sago and buckwheat flour can be used in a variety of ways for cakes, bread, biscuits and pancakes for those who are sensitive to wheat, and recipes can be found in the FORESIGHT *Wholefood Cookbook* by Norman and Ruth Jervis, *Cook Yourself a Favour* by Gibson & Templeton and in *Wheatless Cooking* by Linnette Coffey.

Dove Farm makes an excellent gluten-free mixed flour. Pastry can be made with fine-ground whole-wheat flour, also fine-ground barley and rye flours. Sainsburys and Tesco stock the "Glutofin", "Free From" and "Glutinex" ranges, as do most health stores.

To Be Avoided
White flour and all white flour products such as bread, buns, cakes, scones, biscuits, pasta, white rice and other refined grains, puddings, packet cake and pudding mixes (which also contain sugar and artificial additives) sweets, sweetener, coloured carbonated drinks (some of these contain up to the equivalent of 9 teaspoonfuls of sugar per tin). Most bought jams and jellies which contain a lot of white sugar and artificial colourings and flavourings. For further information on the effects of food additives read the FORESIGHT publication, *Find Out*. In particular, avoid drinks containing Aspartamine, and artificial sweeteners.

Fruit and Vegetables and Vegetable Oils
(Look for Organic at all times)
Dr Weston Price throughout his book, *Nutrition and Physical Degeneration* stressed the advisability of eating fresh raw fruit and vegetables whenever possible. All fruit, fresh, dried or stewed, with or without honey, molasses or a small amount of unrefined sugar is good food. Raw fruit and vegetables can also be chopped or grated for salads. Home bottled fruit should be bottled in water only. It is best to stew fruit in a glass dish or enamel saucepan as the acidity in the juice can leach metal from metal saucepans. Home pressed juices such as blackcurrant, citrus etc are useful to use instead of squash. All juices should be diluted. Many different organic juices are now available, sugar and colouring free.

All fresh vegetables can be safely eaten raw except potatoes and unsprouted pulses. Organically grown vegetables are now available in many greengrocers and supermarkets. A list of local organic growers can be obtained from your Foresight Branch Secretary. The Soil Association organises Box Schemes in many districts. It is a good idea to eat raw salad every day. Salads can contain: whole, chopped or grated lettuce, endive, chicory, white or red cabbage, cress, cauliflower, radish, tomato, cucumber, celery, spring and main crop onions, carrots, button mushrooms, Chinese leaves, watercress, Savoy cabbage, beetroots, small peas, sweet peppers, sprouting seeds and pulses (alfalfa, mung beans and many others are now available in your local health store). Salads can be garnished with nuts, whole or ground, many different herbs, sunflower and sesame seeds, pine kernels, raisins and other dried fruits, dates and grated or chopped fruits of every type.

Dressings can be made of different organic oils and herbs, cider vinegar and lemon juice. Home made mayonnaise, yoghurt, soured cream or Tofu soya bean curd can be used as dressing. Contrasting flavours such as orange in coleslaw can be very nice. Vegetable oils which are available cold pressed (a useful source of Vitamin E and free from the anti-oxidants BHT and BHA) can be used for salad dressings as well as for frying.

When cooking, shallow frying is preferable to deep-fat frying as lower cooking temperatures can be used and less oil is needed. Cooking temperatures should be kept below the point where the oil smokes, a factor which affects the structure of the oil. This change in structure can produce substances that have been found to be carcinogenic. Oil should be used once and then thrown away.

Where cooking vegetables is necessary, methods should be aimed at preserving vitamins and minerals. Potatoes should be baked or steamed in their skins. Vegetables taste better and retain more nutrients scrubbed rather than peeled or scraped. It is possible to buy a stainless steel vegetable steamer that fits into a saucepan and even a triple-decker steamer. This way vegetables can be steamed clear of the water and will retain the most nutrients. Without a steamer, vegetables should be cooked quickly in a little water, and this water should be used for stocks, soups or gravy as it will contain much of the minerals from the vegetables. Vegetables should always be washed quickly and cooked straight away, If they are left soaking in a bowl of water a lot of the nutrients are washed away.

Vegetable juices, carrot, beetroot, celery, tomato etc can be made in a blender. It is also possible to make juices from green leaf vegetables - such as lettuce and cress but these are less attractive visually unless mixed with some more colourful juice such as beetroot. Many vegetable juices are now available bottled and are delicious.

In place of sweets, pieces of carrot, celery, all dried fruits, sunflower seeds, and of course raw fruit can be used for the whole family, once they are old enough to chew thoroughly.

To Be Avoided
Potatoes which have green patches; this indicates a concentration of Solanin which is poisonous. Tinned vegetables which are generally high in salt and may contain sugar and artificial colouring, and which are a poor source of Vitamin C

Unless a potato is diseased it should not be peeled as the vitamin content lies just underneath the skin. Vegetables fried in reheated oil, waterlogged, overcooked, kept warm or reheated will have lost much of the vitamin content, as will vegetables cooked in large amounts of water which is then thrown away. Rhubarb, apple and all acid fruits leach aluminium from the pan (so they are best cooked in enamel pans or glass casseroles in the oven). Fruit tinned in heavy syrup has extra sugar and, in some cases, artificial colouring.

How to Sprout Seeds for Salads
You will need four jars, (clean glass) eg 1lb coffee size, sweet jars or 1.5lb Kilner jars. Remove the lids and replace by a layer of muslin or gauze secured by an elastic band.

Put the seeds to 1/5th of the volume of the jar. Cover with water overnight. Cover with muslin and secure with band, It may not be necessary to remove this until you take out sprouts to eat. In the morning drain through the muslin.

Rinse in cold water and drain again removing as much moisture as possible to permit the air to circulate during the day. Rinse and drain in a similar fashion twice a day.

Once the sprouts are at least as long as the beans or the seeds from which they come, they are ready to eat. They may be eaten whole and raw without further washing.

It takes two to three days for each crop to grow to this stage, after which they are edible for several days more if rinsing and draining is continued. Thus with four jars it is possible to have one each of several different seeds ready to eat at any time. As one jar comes ready another should be started to maintain a continuous supply.

Meat (Organic at all times)

Fresh lean meat, liver, heart, kidney, sweetbreads, tongues, all poultry and game, and fish, especially roe and shellfish are nutritious foods. Meat should be bought as fresh as possible. Organic, free-range poultry is now available from many shops and farms. Venison, rabbit, game birds, pigeon and all seafoods are especially good foods as usually the animals have been in their natural environment and not intensively farmed. Mutton, lamb and offal from sheep is usually less intensively farmed than beef, pork and poultry.

Meat is best roasted, grilled or stewed with stock and vegetables. The stock will then contain much of the goodness in the form of nutrients and flavouring from the meat, and can be eaten as meat soup, or gravy and not thrown away. Some butchers will make sausages free from preservatives and other additives on request. Bone broth made from simmering joint bones, poultry carcasses etc is a useful source of minerals. This can be used to make any form of soup.

Since FORESIGHT was formed a great many more farmers have decided to adopt organic methods, and as a result free-range poultry and eggs are much more widely available. Supermarkets now stock organic produce. Where the organic produce tends to be higher in cost, this is because of smaller scale production, more attention paid to better quality feedstuffs and the avoidance of using hormones and poly-phosphates.

The cooked organically-raised chicken is particularly good value compared with its battery-produced counterpart, as the free-range bird has less shrinkage, more flavour and better texture.

To Be Avoided

Meat fried in reheated fat, meat kept warm for long periods, twice cooked meat. Tinned meats which contain sodium nitrate (E250 and E251). Commercial pates, bacon, sausages, packet ham etc which contain preservatives and sometimes the flavour-enhancer monosodium glutamate (621), Commercial sauces for meat may contain monosodium glutamate (621) sugar and colourings. All meat from animals fed extra hormones and antibiotics (ie all non-organic meat!).

(Non-organic beef has added estrogens which are female hormones. Hormones are used to artificially accelerate growth and the poly-phosphates to enable water to be held in suspension in the muscles of the meat giving a pseudo increased plumpness to the carcass. Whether these are harmful or not has been much debated and much of the controversy has been reproduced in the vegetarian book, *Why You Don't Need Meat* by Peter Cox, Thorsons 1986. I think the arguments are certainly forceful on why we don't need intensively produced meat!)

Dairy Products and Eggs (Organic at all times)

Fresh whole milk, butter, cheese, cream and yoghurt is good food for those who are not sensitive to bovine products. Unpasteurised goat's milk from healthy TT accredited herds is again available in supermarkets. This is a useful source of B complex vitamins (including B2 which is otherwise destroyed by pasteurisation, as is the amino acid lysine) and contains digestive enzymes which can improve the digestibility of milk for some people. All milk should be stored, covered, in a refrigerator to prevent bacterial contamination.

Skimmed or semi-skimmed milk is available which has had the fat wholly or partially removed. Although the calcium content remains the same, there will be a loss of the fat-soluble vitamins A and D, of which milk is usually an important source. Skimmed and semi-skimmed milks should not be used for children under twelve years of age - if fat intake is a concern, avoid fatty meats, fried meats, fried foods and hidden sources of fat in cakes, biscuits and ice cream. Cheese and butter are good foods except those containing preservatives and artificial colourings (check labels). Goat's milk and cheese, and goat's and sheep's yoghurt are widely available and these may be very useful where people are sensitive to cow's milk. Delicious milk shakes can be made with goat's milk and honey. ("The Land of Milk and Honey" was, of course, the land of goat's milk and honey!). Fresh ice cream can be made with fresh cream, eggs and honey and if wished, flavoured with fruit puree. Home-made cream cheese can be made using herbs. Goat's milk is however a poor source of folic acid so if you are using goat's milk exclusively be sure to include a daily source of folate in the form of leafy green veg (see other sources in Vitamin List at the end of this leaflet.)

Supermarkets are providing organic free range eggs, so obtaining these should no longer be a problem, and duck, goose and guinea fowl eggs add variety, as do quail eggs in season.

Milk can be used in cooking in sweet or savoury sauces and in soup. Also: sago pudding, tapioca pudding, cornflour pudding, whole, flaked or ground brown rice pudding, whole or cracked millet pudding, semolina, junket, milk jelly with fresh fruit puree, fruit souffle, fruit fools with fresh fruit puree, egg custard.

For those with milk allergy rice milk is available which may be a useful alternative. It is important to include alternative sources of protein, calcium and vitamins A and D. Green vegetables, dolomite tablets and fish liver oils should be used daily.

To Be Avoided.
Tinned evaporated milk. Dried milks, as drying destroys nutrients such as Vitamin B2, arachidonic acid and lysine. Yoghurts and flavoured milk drinks if they contain artificial flavourings, colourings and preservatives.

General Comments
Since 1978 when FORESIGHT was formed, the dietary advice outlined here has been confirmed as beneficial both by scientific research and by the happy experience of FORESIGHT members.

The increasing trend towards organic agriculture in the last few years has brought foods free from hazards of contamination or deficiency to a much wider public. At the same time many people are starting to grow their own vegetables and fruit organically, and surplus may be available for swapping or selling locally. Farmer's markets are beginning to make a comeback. Allotments are becoming fashionable again. Many fruit trees are very ornamental as well as functional and people enjoy having one or more in their garden. (It is necessary to choose a self-fertilising variety if there is only room for one, - or share a plan with neighbour!). Town dwellers can have highly successful roof gardens or balconies where cultivation can take place in tubs, troughs and plastic bags! For the beginner in organic gardening Lawrence Hills excellent little book *Organic Gardening* can be obtained from The Henry Doubleday Research Association, Ryton-in-Dunsmore, Coventry, Warwickshire. It is well worth joining the HDRA or the Good Gardener's Association, who exist to help people learn how to grow food organically. See Useful Addresses pages 213 to 216.

The importance of trace elements from food sources is becoming clearer with each decade, as research in these areas becomes more sophisticated. It is possible that food factors associated with nutrient absorption are yet to be discovered. Basing the diet on fresh whole foods grown on healthy soil appears to be a sensible way to help to ensure optimum nutritional status.

For many people however, convenience foods are still a part of the diet, and many of these foods have been stored for some time before they reach the consumer. Similarly, custom dictates that food such as meat is cooked and milk is pasteurised. The result of this practice is nutrient loss Therefore it is not surprising that dietary deficiencies can occur. Add to this the fact that much food is raised on poor soil lacking in essential trace minerals, after years in which crops have been raised with the use of artificial fertilisers, and it is easy to see average food sources may not be ideal!

Many prospective parents suffer from mild allergic conditions, intestinal parasites or candida albicans. Some may have absorption that has been impaired by over-consumption of wheat and cow's milk. Those who have been eating many white flour and sugar products may have very poor levels of trace minerals. Copper and lead from water and dust may also have reduced levels of trace minerals.

Add to this the individual's increased need for extra high levels of specific nutrients in times of stress and at specific times of life such as infancy, teething, adolescence, pregnancy, lactation, old age and while endeavouring to procreate, the quality of the food sources in terms of nutrient content and freedom from artificial additives, becomes a vital factor in the maintenance of health. Foetal integrity and paternal and maternal nutrition is closely linked. This has been borne out by animal experiments, by epidemiological studies and by the experience of many FORESIGHT couples.

FORESIGHT's nutritional advisors have helped to formulate the well-balanced supplements of vitamins and trace minerals, which, taken in conjunction with the diet as described, has proved very helpful. We are aware that many people feel that a "good diet supplies all the vitamins and minerals necessary", but from the beginning we have favoured the "belt and braces" approach and have seen nothing to contradict this view down the years. In fact in 2003 I think we have the experience behind us to be able to say beyond doubt that the supplements do contribute to the health of our babies *and their parents!*

I do not feel qualified to give a run down of all the **ethical** considerations of every packet on the shelves. However, on a personal level, I am trying to take on board the morality (as well as the nutritional value, the gluten content, the compatibility with the environment, and so on!) of what goes into my basket.

As they begin to make this *easier* for us by more explicit labelling, I am sure, good-hearted, label-reading crowd that we are, we will be doing our best to be ethical as well as toxin-free and cheerfully well-nourished!

SOME CHARTS SHOWING THE RELEVANCE OF NUTRITIONAL STATUS

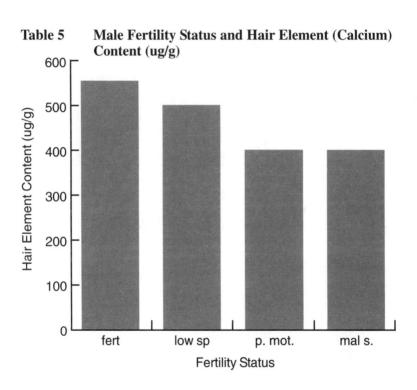

Table 5 **Male Fertility Status and Hair Element (Calcium) Content (ug/g)**

Key	
fert	fertile
low sp	low sperm count
p. mot.	poor motility
mal s	malformed sperm

Table 6 **Male Fertility Status and Hair Element (Magnesium) Content (ug/g)**

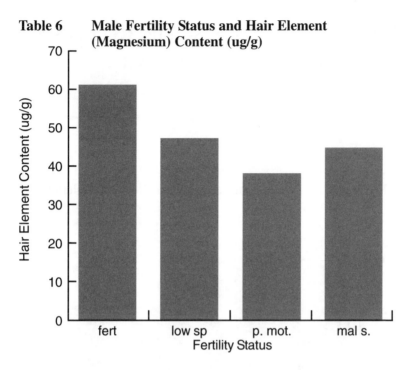

Table 7 **Male Fertility Status and Hair Element (Potassium) Content (ug/g)**

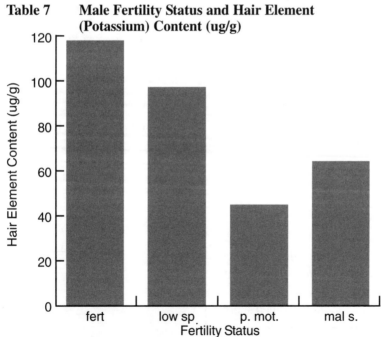

Table 8 **Male Fertility Status and Hair Element (Zinc) Content (ug/g)**

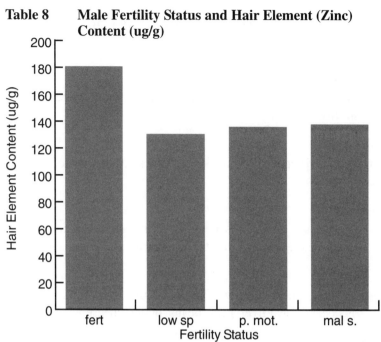

Table 9 **Male Fertility Status and Hair Element (Selenium) Content (ug/g)**

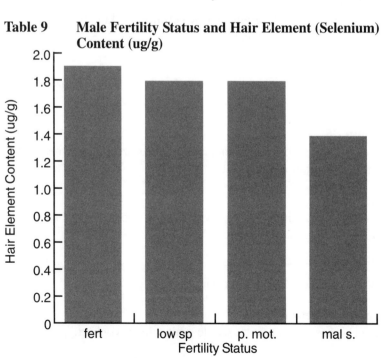

VITAMINS AND MINERALS - DIETARY SOURCES

Vitamin A
Milk, butter, cheese, yoghurt, egg yolk, liver, kidneys, sweetbreads, fatty fish, fish liver oil.

Carotene
Carrot, bean, red pepper, broccoli, kale, chard, spinach, tomato, marrow, apricot, peaches.

Vitamin B1
Whole grains, nuts, dried beans, peas, lentils, soya beans, peanut butter, liver, kidney, heart, brewer's yeast, wheat germ, pork, ham, eggs.

Vitamin B2
Brewer's yeast, wheat germ, whole grains, green veg, milk, yoghurt, eggs, soya beans, meat liver, peas, beans, butter, cheese.

Nicotinamide
Brewer's yeast, whole grain, wheat germ, liver, kidneys, green veg, fish, potato, nuts, eggs, meat.

Pantothenic Acid
Brewer's yeast, whole grains, wheat germ, liver, kidney, heart, mushrooms, yeast, green veg.

Vitamin B6
Brewer's yeast, whole grains, molasses, liver, heart, kidney, wheat germ, peanuts, mushrooms, potatoes.

Folic Acid
Brewer's yeast, whole grains, liver, kidney, green veg, wheat germ, milk.

Vitamin B12
Milk, eggs, cheese, meat, liver, kidney, fish.

Para-amino-benzoic acid
Brewer's yeast, wheat germ, whole grains, liver, yoghurt.

Biotin
Brewer's yeast, mushrooms, milk, eggs, liver, kidneys, heart.

Choline
Brewer's yeast, whole grains, wheat germ, liver, meat, eggs, green veg, legumes.

Inositol
Brewer's yeast, whole grains, wheat germ, liver, meat, eggs, green veg, legumes.

Vitamin C
Oranges, lemons, grapefruits, tangerines, clementines, satsumas, ugli fruit, wilkins, limes, blackcurrants, rose hips, strawberries, raspberries, guavas, bananas, apples, mangoes, nectarines, melons, pears, plums, peaches, apricots, grapes, peppers, pimentos, cabbage, carrot, cauliflower, potatoes, peas, Brussels sprouts, spinach, kale, beans, watercress, cress, endives, cucumbers, chicory, lettuces, beetroots, sprouting seeds, swede, parsley, pineapple.

Vitamin D
Sunshine, milk, butter, eggs, fortified margarine, fatty fish, fish liver oil.

Vitamin E
Unrefined oils (cold pressed), whole grains, wheat germ, milk, egg yolk, green leafy vegetables, lettuce, avocado, nuts, seeds, nut butter (cold pressed).

EFAs (Essential Fatty Acids)
Unrefined oils, nuts, nut butters, green leafy veg, seeds, fatty fish.

Calcium
Milk, cheese, bone broth, green veg, egg, dolomite, bone meal.

Magnesium
Milk, eggs, green veg, seafood, whole grains, dolomite.

Potassium
Whole grains, wheat germ, soya flour, nuts, all fresh fruit, all vegetables.

Copper
Whole grains, liver, kidney, brain, green veg.

Iron
Lean meats, liver, apricots, eggs, kidneys, whole grains, molasses, eggs, shellfish, dried fruits.

Manganese
Whole grains, wheat germ, seeds, leafy veg, brewer's yeast, egg, liver, onions, green beans, parsley, strawberries, bananas, apples, pineapple, cherries.

Zinc
Whole grains, brewer's yeast, wheat germ, all fruit, all vegetables, nuts, offal, meat, fish, poultry, shellfish.

Chromium
Brewer's yeast, whole grains, wheat germ, fruits, vegetables, black pepper, beef, liver, beets, molasses, beer, mushrooms.

Selenium
Brewer's yeast, whole grains, garlic, liver, eggs.

Cobalt
Brewer's yeast, whole grains, meat, liver, nuts, fruit, vegetables.

Nickel
Grains, vegetables.

Vanadium
Black pepper, soya bean oil, corn oil, olive oil, olives, gelatine.

Iodine
Water, seafish, iodised salt, watercress, onions, kelp, shellfish.

REASONS FOR TRACE MINERAL DEFICIENCIES

So let us look closely at all the reasons for poor nutrient status that beset us today, quite apart from just poor food choice, or the ubiquitous "slimming" regimes, coupled to an exhausting life-style!

- **Antibiotics**
  (destroy beneficial gut flora which aid absorption and encourage overgrowth of candida)

- **Copper and Lead Piping**
  (contaminated water gives toxic intake which reduces micronutrients)

- **Excess Chlorine in drinking water**
  (can destroy/impair development of intestinal flora)

- **Refined Carbohydrates, white flour and sugar**
  (lack basic nutrients)

- **White Sugar**
  (leaches nutrients needed to metabolise it as it contains virtually none)

- **Na/K/P fertilisers**
  (impoverish soil as they do not replace lost trace minerals)

- **Zinc-Phosphate bonding**
  (caused by Na/K/P fertilisers, makes zinc less available to plants)

- **Herbicides Landing On Top Of The Soil**
  (kill the micro-bacteria that would provide protein to facilitate the uptake of micronutrients such as manganese)

- **Contraceptive Pill**
  (reduces zinc, manganese and magnesium)
  (+Clomid etc) (reduces zinc and magnesium)

- **Infection/Injury/Surgery**
  (requires zinc for healing)

- **Organophosphates**
  (inhibit uptake of manganese from the gut)

- **Smoking, Alcohol, Drugs**
  (squander zinc, selenium, vitamins A and E, and cobalt and chromium)

- **Specific Food Additives**
  (lower levels of zinc and magnesium)

- **Stress**
  (lowers levels of zinc and B complex vitamins)

- **Scraping down old leaded paints**
  (contaminates with lead, which reduces micronutrients and calcium)

- **Allergic illness**
  (can overstimulate immune system and squander zinc, and can cause malabsorption and sometimes diarrhoea inhibiting absorption of all nutrients)

- **Gut parasites**
  (squander all nutrients by helping themselves to your food!)

So, the food is inadequate to start with, and there are lots of environmental factors making it all worse!

Now, let's have a look at what we do about it all:

. . . .

MAIN PRINCIPLES OF NUTRITIONAL PROGRAMME

Organic Whole Grain Foods

Organic Full Proteins (Meat, Poultry, Fish)

Organic Vegetables and Fruit, (preferably raw except for potatoes and red beans)

Organic Eggs and Dairy Products

Avoid White Flour and Sugar

Avoid Excess Tea, Coffee

Avoid Excess Canned and Packet Foods

Avoid Hazardous Additives

Golden Rules
(how to remember!)

1. Organic. Whenever you can. Think Green!

2. No refined carbohydrates. Think Brown!

3. No hazardous additives. Think Colour free!

4. Filter the water. Think Transparent!

• • • • • • • • • • • • • • • • • • •

Basis of Balanced Diet
(another memory aid)

Fruits and vegetables, raw, cooked, dried & juiced, soy, nuts & nut butters **5**	Meat, poultry, offal, fish, game, shellfish, molluscs **2**
4 Grains, whole or crushed, raw or cooked, Rice dream	**3** Dairy produce, cow, goat & sheep, eggs, hen, goose, duck & quail

The figures in the corners of the square indicate a good number of servings per day for that particular food group.

These are just for guidance, not to be followed slavishly!

SUGGESTIONS TO BE CONSIDERED FOR DAILY MENUS

Breakfast
Whole carbohydrates, bread* or cereals, fruit, fruit juice, yoghurts. If preferred, cooked breakfast: fried bread or potatoes/mushrooms, tomatoes, bananas, or prunes/bacon, egg, fish, sausage, etc. Fry in a small amount of oil or grill.

Lunch (if main meal)
Meat, poultry, fish, offal, sausage etc. Potatoes rice, polenta or pasta. 2 vegetables, 1 root, 1 green. Dairy & fruit dessert, or cheese and fruit. Sponge, pancakes, crumble or pastry puddings made with whole-grain flours.

Lunch (if secondary meal)
Whole-wheat protein sandwich: (ham, egg, sardine, salmon, nut butter, cheese, tongue, corned beef, chicken etc with salad). Fruit & yoghurt or cheese.

Tea (if major meal)
Hot soup. Cold meats and salad. Fish & chips. (Grilled tomatoes, baked beans) Wholegrain cakes, biscuits, bread*, pancakes. Dairy pudding and fruit, nuts, dried fruits. Sponge or pastry puddings made with whole-grain flours. Whole-wheat biscuits & cheese.

Tea (if snack meal)
Whole-wheat bread*, cakes, scones, biscuits. Juice, herb tea, milk, rice or soy substitute, or soup, or yoghurt. Dried or fresh fruits or nuts, or salad.

Dinner/Supper (if main meal) see Lunch given above.

Dinner/Supper (if snack meal) from sample menus given above.

*Alternate butter with oil-based spreads. Use nut butters, goat's cheese, honey, sugar-free jams and jellies. Marmite and similar yeast spreads - if yeast is not a problem.

Avoid processed, tinned and packet foods, microwaved foods, excess tea and coffee and ersatz drinks with sugar substitutes and artificial colouring and flavourings, confectionery and white flour products.

"Eat Organic" whenever possible.

PRACTICAL TIPS FOR THE KITCHEN

1. Eat food fresh. Avoid storing fruit and vegetables wherever possible. Where inevitable, store in a cool place.
2. Avoid preparing in advance.
3. Use mineral water for boiling and use for soups or gravy.
4. Do not overcook. Heat destroys B complex vitamins and vitamin C.
5. Do not cook at all if it can be eaten raw! (You can graze mustard and cress!)
6. Make bread with yeast. Shop-bought bread (made with bicarbonate of soda) contains phytates which interfere with the absorption of zinc and calcium. Raising the dough with yeast inactivates the phytates.
7. Soak muesli in the fridge overnight to destroy phytates. Phytates prevent the absorption of vital minerals such as calcium and zinc.
8. Boil the water first and add vegetables to minimise oxidation and loss of vitamin C, or preferably steam them.
9. Serve foods promptly after cooking.
10. Use stainless steel, enamelled or glass cookware. Aluminium is a toxic substance which accumulates in the body
11. Grill rather than fry food, if frying, use oil rather than hard fats. (Discard oil after use). Stir frying in a minimum of oil is the frying method of choice.
12. Many vegetables can be braised in the oven in a closed dish, moistened with stock.
13. Avoid microwaved foods, as this can destroy vitamins and enzymes in the food.
14. Filter all drinking water and cooking water, or use bottled water
15. Use milk from cartons rather than bottles, as the light destroys Vitamin B2.
16. Avoid hazardous colourings and other food chemicals.
17. Use eggs from free range hens, preferably organically fed.
18. Peas, beans and lentils and the pectin from apples are natural ways of increasing the elimination of toxic metals.

CONCENTRATED NUTRIENT SOURCES

Alfalfa and mung bean sprouted seeds
Black molasses, and honey
Brewer's Yeast products
Cold-pressed safflower, sunflowers and linseed oils
Goat & sheep milk yoghurts, natural live yoghurt
Spirulina
Wheatgerm (for those who can tolerate wheat)

Filter Drinking and Cooking Water

(To Avoid Lead, Pesticides, Nitrates, Estrogens and Excess Chlorine and Copper).

Pesticides, fluorides and estrogens need to be avoided. Tap water is possibly treated with fluoride which has well documented health risks, including increasing the risk of cancer and Down's Syndrome. Fluoride in toothpaste makes gums bleed and causes mouth ulcers. (Find one without. There are Kingfisher's, Tom's and Aloe Vera toothpastes in the health stores and some supermarkets.) As of going to press, the Government are threatening us with fluoride in different areas. I would find out from your local water authority every few months what they are doing. At the same time, tell them that you do not want it. If they are using it, my advice would be to use bottled water. Fluoride passes through all the water filters out there. *Unfortunately there is no way they can get fluoride out of the reservoirs once they have put it in.* If there is fluoride in your area, drink bottled water. Hopefully, most of the bottled waters are not contaminated.

In addition to the fluoride problems I am not happy with the water. If the fish are changing sex in it, why should we be happy? It is better not to drink tap water while trying to procreate. It is said to be frequently high in estrogens - this is highly disadvantageous to sperm.

The water can leach metal from the pipes and often contains high levels of copper and, less frequently, of lead. In rural areas there may be pesticides, herbicides, sheep dip and nitrates. High levels of chlorine used to eliminate harmful bacteria may compromise the gut flora (bugs in your intestine which help the digestion of food).

Apart from these disadvantages, (which are bad enough!) there might be genetically modified pollen in the wind falling on surface water. We do not know enough about genetic modification.

So how is your tap-water today?
Are we all breathing in the fall-out from the pollen of the flowers from the strawberry whose mother went for a walk with a fish? Will this prove to be bothersome at some future date? Should we try and impress it upon Those Who Rule that we would rather not have the possibility made available to us until they find exactly what this does to the bees, butterflies, birds and *definitely to us*? When they have found out, will they kindly tell us, and let us assist them in their deliberations, rather than keep it from us and make dubious decisions on our behalf? At the moment Monsanto seems to be retreating but we need to watch the situation.

So we suggest the Boots jug water filter to use for drinking and cooking water - if they are not fluoridated. It is the easy and cheap way to remove about two thirds of the pollutants. These filters can be obtained from Boots for about £20.00, at time of going to press. Otherwise, there are a number of "whole house" filters which also gives a clean bath or shower. See useful addresses for Freshwater Filters.

If a tap water test reveals very high levels of copper or lead, I would get a whole house filter fitted, as metals can be absorbed from the bathwater.

If your area is fluoridated it seems we have to fall back on bottled water which is expensive and heavy to carry home. Tell your MP how you feel about this, also your water company, and your local council, who may be asking them to put it in.

You get the message?

We are not just about "getting a pregnancy" at FORESIGHT. Our long-term objective is a normal, healthy baby, with his full physical and mental potential unimpaired. This is why we go to all this trouble to get it right and to get him a sound, healthy environment to grow up in.

Here follows the chart from Rutger's University to explain why we say "eat organic".

Table 10 Variations in mineral content in vegetables
(Firman E Baer Report, Rutgers University)

	% of dry weight		Milequivalents per 100g dry weight				Trace elements (parts per million dry matter)				
	Total ash or mineral content	Phosphorus	Calcium	Magnesium	Potassium	Sodium	Boron	Manganese	Iron	Copper	Cobalt
SNAP BEANS											
Organic	10.45	0.36	40.50	60.00	99.70	8.60	73.00	60.00	227.00	69.00	0.26
Inorganic	4.04	0.22	15.50	14.80	29.10	0.00	10.00	2.00	10.00	3.00	0.00
CABBAGE											
Organic	10.38	0.38	60.00	43.60	148.30	20.40	42.00	13.00	94.00	48.00	0.15
Inorganic	6.12	0.18	17.50	15.60	53.70	0.80	7.00	2.00	20.00	0.40	0.00
LETTUCE											
Organic	24.48	0.43	71.00	49.30	176.50	12.20	37.00	169.00	516.00	60.00	0.19
Inorganic	7.01	0.22	16.00	13.10	53.70	0.00	6.00	1.00	9.00	3.00	0.00
TOMATOES											
Organic	14.20	0.35	23.00	59.20	148.30	6.50	36.00	68.00	1,938.00	53.00	0.63
Inorganic	6.07	0.16	4.50	4.50	58.80	0.00	5.00	1.00	1.00	0.00	0.00
SPINACH											
Organic	28.50	0.52	96.00	203.90	257.00	69.50	88.00	117.00	1,584.00	32.00	0.25
Inorganic	12.38	0.27	47.50	46.90	64.60	0.80	12.00	1.00	19.00	0.50	0.20

ORGANIC is better for you!

Aspartame etc

Another ubiquitous health hazard is the prevalence of a group of additives known as "excitotoxins". These include the following:

Monosodium glutamate
Aspartame/Aspartate/Aspartic acid
Cysteine/L-Cysteine
Hydrolysed Protein/Hydrolysed Vegetable Protein
Glutamine/Glutamic acid
Kainate
Natural Flavouring
NMDA
Nutri sweet
Phenylalanine
Quisqualate
Sodium Caseinate
Textured Protein
Autolyzed Yeast
Bouillon
Broth
Flavouring
Malt Extract
Malt Flavouring
Natural Beef or Chicken Flavouring
Natural Flavouring
Seasoning
Spices
Stock
Carrageenan
Enzymes
Soy Protein Concentrate
Whey Protein Concentrate

They can produce a cluster of symptoms that mimic those of a brain tumour - severe headaches, dizziness, and loss of peripheral vision, even in bad cases really worrying loss of eye-sight. Quite often patients have quite an anxious few weeks waiting for tests on our hard pressed NHS, before discovering that all will be well if they just stop using the foods that contain these additives.

Other symptoms that can crop up if you are particularly unlucky include:

> Alzheimer's
> Atrophy, developmental failure of the sexual organs
> Autism
> Brain damage (sometimes delayed onset)
> Cerebral palsy
> Degenerative diseases
> Diabetes
> Dyslexia
> Epilepsy
> Endocrine damage
> Eye damage
> Foetal damage
> Hypoglycaemia
> Hyperactivity
> Impaired growth
> Insomnia
> Low thyroid function
> Lowered fertility
> Lowered intelligence
> Migraine
> Obesity
> Placental damage
> Schizophrenia
> Sexual psychopathology
> Sudden rages

Examine the labels of fizzy drinks, sweets, pre-cooked meals, and all "diet" foods that proudly announce they are "Sugar Free". You will find one of the aliases of aspartame. Look especially at Chinese foods, and cheap prepared meals for MSG. The longer a food is expected to sit on a shelf, the more the flavour can be expected to "fade", and the more these artificial "aids" will be brought into play.

Once again . . . read the labels!

Table 11

Safe Additives Agreed by One and All
(E Millstone, M Hanssen, The London Food Alliance)

Colourings - Yellow

E100	E101 (i)	E101 (ii)

Colourings - Green

E140 (i)	E140 (ii)

Colourings - Plant Extracts

E160 (a)(i)	E160 (a)(ii)	E160 (b)	E160 (c)	E160 (e)
E160 (f)	E161	E161 (a)	E161 (c)	E 161(d)
E161 (e)	E161 (f)	E161 (g)	E162	E163

Other Colourings

E170	E172

Preservatives

E234	E260	E262 (i)	E263	E297

Antioxidants

E301	E302	E304	E306	E307
E308	E309			

Emulsifiers etc.

E322	E331	E331 (i)	E331 (ii)	E331(iii)
E335 (i)	E335 (ii)	E337	E350	E350 (i)
E350 (ii)	E351	E352	E352 (i)	E352 (ii)
E353	E355	E363	E375	E400
E401	E402	E404	E405	E440 (b)

Acids, Bases and Related Materials

E501	E501 (i)	E501 (ii)	E503	E503 (i)
E516 (i)				

Anticaking Agents etc.

E551	E552	E576	E577	E578

CHAPTER 4

SMOKING, ALCOHOL AND STREET DRUGS

Our advice is very simple - don't!

Tobacco smoke and alcohol are both significant toxins in their own right, and the health of the whole planet would bound ahead if they were eliminated once and for all! However, we live in an imperfect world, and huge amounts of money are involved, so poisonous and addictive substances will continue to be available and seductively presented so that those who produce them can lift our money off us in a gigantic way!

Apart from the factor of the toxin itself, there is the serious squandering of the nutrients that are involved with removing it from the body or protecting the relevant tissues.

Smoking squanders selenium, Vitamins A, E and C, (needed to protect lung tissue), and good old zinc, which is always called for when healing is needed. Nicotine is also a toxic substance that acts on sperm as a poison. Tobacco also contains cadmium and lead both of which are foeto-toxic. Alcohol squanders zinc (needed to activate the enzyme alcohol dehydrogenase) and all the B-complex vitamins, especially B12, and Vitamin C, iron, and also chromium that is particularly needed for sugar metabolism. It is also a toxin that reduces spermatogenesis and sperm motility in its own right.

> Thus, they each present a double whammy to sperm health and a quadruple whammy if you use both!

Chronic alcoholism can induce atrophy of the testicle, and this is well documented. Even at a lower intake, alcohol can cause deterioration in sperm concentration, output and motility (eagerness to reach the ova!) There is nothing macho about poisoned shrivelled testicles!

These are some bar charts from the FORESIGHT Study at the University of Surrey demonstrating how alcohol interferes with iron metabolism as does smoking, and the effect this has on male fertility status. Further charts show the response of zinc status to smoking and alcohol activity and the effect on the fertility of the man.

A further chart shows the relationship of cadmium concentration in the hair following smoking and the effect cadmium has on lowering male fertility. Note also the effect that lead levels have on male fertility.

Table 12   Hair Iron Concentration and Smoking Activity

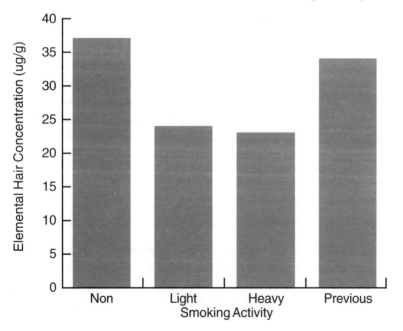

Table 13 **Hair Iron Concentration and Alcohol Consumption**

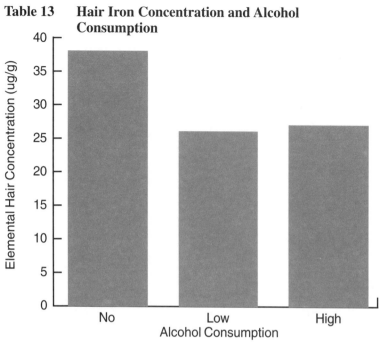

Table 14 **Male Fertility Status and Hair Element (Iron) Content (ug/g)**

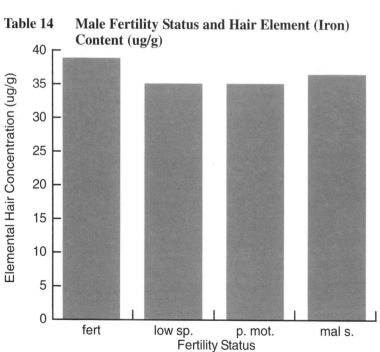

Table 15   Hair Zinc Concentration and Smoking Activity

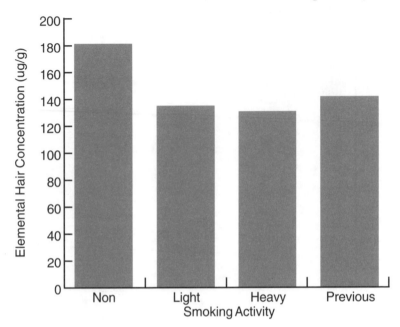

Table 16   Male Hair Zinc Concentration and Alcohol Consumption

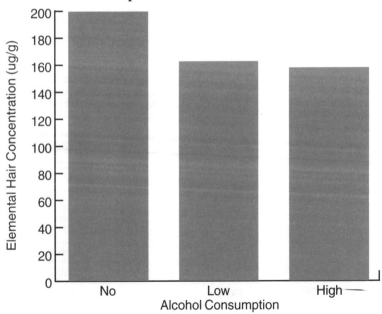

Table 17   Male Fertility Status and Hair Element (Zinc) Content (ug/g)

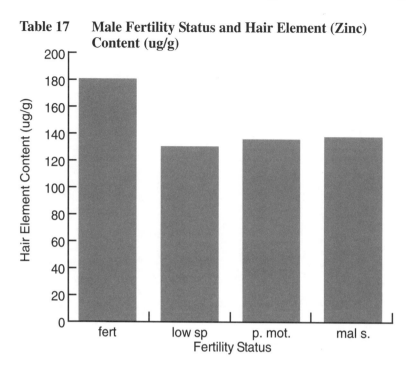

Table 18   Hair Cadmium Concentration and Smoking Activity

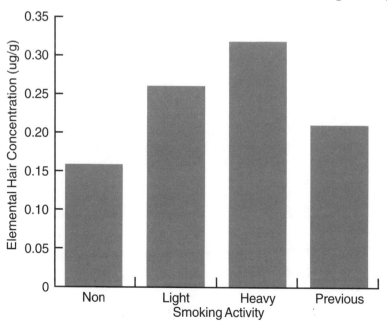

Table 19   Male Fertility Status and Hair Element (Cadmium) Content (ug/g)

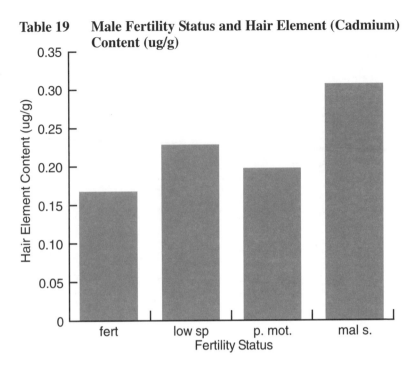

Table 20   Male Fertility Status and Hair Element (Lead) Content (ug/g)

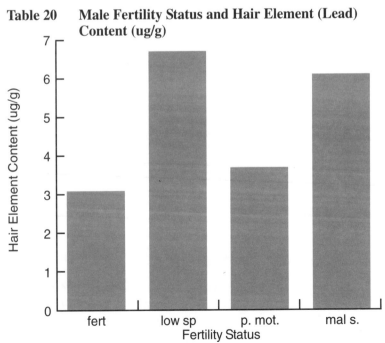

TYPICAL CHARTS REGARDING MALE INFERTILITY

Two typical hair analysis charts follow. Chart A of a man who smoked 105 cigarettes a week and had 60 drinks, and whose wife had suffered two miscarriages followed by two and a half years of infertility.

	Your Results	**Recommended Values**	
Calcium:	286.00	400.00	mg/kg
Magnesium:	42.00	35.00	mg/kg
Potassium:	81.00	75.00	mg/kg
Iron:	36.00	30.00	mg/kg
Chromium:	0.73	0.8	mg/kg
Cobalt:	0.23	0.25	mg/kg
Copper:	21.00	20.00	mg/kg
Manganese:	3.42	1.5	mg/kg
Nickel:	0.92	0.8	mg/kg
Selenium:	1.64	2.25	mg/kg
Zinc:	148.00	185.00	mg/kg
		Threshold Values	
Aluminium:	3.14	2.5	mg/kg
Cadmium:	1.14	0.25	mg/kg
Mercury:	0.22	0.4	mg/kg
Lead:	3.72	1.0	mg/kg

Small wonder when you look at the much reduced Calcium, Chromium, Selenium and Zinc, and the burden of toxic metals. Cadmium comes almost entirely from smoking.

NB Normal values on these two charts were those pertaining to the Finnigans instrument at the University of Surrey.

Chart B records the levels of a man with 75% abnormal sperm attending an alcohol correction unit. He was also a smoker. Note the low levels of zinc and selenium and high levels of toxic metals denoting impaired liver and kidney function.

	Your Results	**Recommended Values**	
Calcium:	412.00	400.00	mg/kg
Magnesium:	37.00	35.00	mg/kg
Potassium:	83.00	75.00	mg/kg
Iron:	49.00	30.00	mg/kg
Chromium:	0.74	0.8	mg/kg
Cobalt:	0.23	0.25	mg/kg
Copper:	22.00	20.00	mg/kg
Manganese:	1.83	1.5	mg/kg
Nickel:	0.72	0.8	mg/kg
Selenium:	1.23	2.25	mg/kg
Zinc:	157.00	185.00	mg/kg
		Threshold Values	
Aluminium:	3.18	2.5	mg/kg
Cadmium:	0.11	0.25	mg/kg
Mercury:	0.08	0.4	mg/kg
Lead:	4.93	1.0	mg/kg

Again, note the low Chromium, Nickel, Selenium, and Zinc, and the high level of Lead. Zinc is particularly necessary for sperm development, and selenium is needed for sperm motility.

In our booklet, *The Adverse Effects of Alcohol on Reproduction,* Tuula Tuormaa has this to say:

> *"Alcohol is a direct testicular toxin. It causes atrophy of semeniferous tubules, loss of sperm cells, and an increase in abnormal sperm. Alcohol is also known to be a strong Leydig cell toxin, and it can have an adverse effect on the synthesis and secretion of testosterone. Alcohol can cause significant deterioration of sperm concentration, sperm output and motility. Semen samples of men consuming excessive amounts of alcohol have shown distinct morphological abnormalities. It has been also established that approximately 80% of chronic alcoholic men are sterile and, furthermore, that alcohol is one of the most common causes of male impotence."*

A lot has been written on the disadvantages to the foetus of maternal drinking, (which are manifold), but comparatively little has been researched regarding the effects of the father's alcohol consumption. However, I make no apologies for assuming that a substance that can destroy sperm heads, atrophy seminal tubules and can curtail the integrity and motility of the sperm produced, will be doing no good at all to the health of the sperm!

Spermatogenesis takes 116 days - the creation of the sperm from Day 1 in the sperm bed, to the day when it sallies forth on its momentous trip. One could think of this almost as a dress rehearsal for the pregnancy. The sperm needs to be cosseted and cared for to reach optimum health at maturity. No drugs, no toxins, no bugs, no deficiencies of the essential nutrients, a perfect environment produces a perfect sperm.

It is all a part of a long continuum of love - 116 days to make a strong and viable sperm - 40 weeks of support within the womb to make a happy healthy baby emerge into the world, 5 years of home environment to make a confident little school child, 21 years of bringing-up and providing for, to see the emergence of a well-balanced young adult. Quite a long haul really, but what is more worth doing?

Smoking

Smoking in men has been linked to a decrease in sperm density (not so many to the amount of fluid produced), a lower proportion of sperm moving well, a decreased sperm count overall, and a reduced output of testosterone (male hormone). Also, there is a higher output of abnormal sperm, which has been directly linked to abnormalities in the subsequent babies. Gustavson KH et al from Sweden, studying the origins of severe mental abnormality indicated that 35% of mental subnormalities could be attributable to chromosomal abnormalities linked to male smoking. What a burden could have been replaced by joy for all the families of the handicapped if this fact had been more widely known and more frequently acted upon.

Happily, there is quite a lot of help at hand for those who are somewhat daunted by the thought of life without a drag and a glass of booze!

In *Prescription for Nutritional Healing* by Balch and Balch, Avery Publishing Group, the following nutrients are recommended for people who have difficulty giving up alcohol:

Vitamins of the B-complex, especially Vitamin B12 and Nicotinamide, Essential fatty acids, L-glutamine, L-methionine, Magnesium, Pantothenate, Vitamin C with Bioflavanoids, Lecithin, Selenium, Choline and Vitamins A, D and E.

I would also include zinc! This is not as exacting as it may seem, as all the vitamins can be found in a comprehensive multivitamin. The oils can be bought as a liquid or capsules and the Calcium, Magnesium and Zinc will all be present in a good multi-mineral. Extra B and Zinc, which may be helpful in the early weeks, can be obtained individually. If the liver is struggling (you feel very low), extra Vitamin C will also help, as will a herbal preparation called HEP 194 from Biocare. Your hair analysis from Foresight will mean you have a tailor made programme, advising on exactly what you need.

The recommendations for the aspiring non-smoker are much of the same, but Balch and Balch would add extra B12 and folic acid, also even larger doses of Vitamins A and E, and selenium. Again, Vitamin C to help clear the liver is a top priority.

Cleansing the toxins out of the system and restoring the body's natural vitality as quickly as possible will make quitting much easier. So may using some form of alternative therapy as a support factor. Reflexology, acupuncture, hypnosis and homeopathy are all out there. The "company" of a therapist battling alongside you and the added motivation may be another factor. See Annex 1 for useful addresses to find help of this kind.

Strategies for Giving Up
Smoking - Nicotine patches are said to be helpful in the first few weeks, but it is important not to wear a nicotine patch *and* smoke! This gives you (and the sperm beds) a double dose. Patches must be used very responsibly.

Some people find it easiest to give up gradually, giving up the first cigarette of the day by saying to themselves "later!" Each "smoke time" is moved on once a week. (But if you smoke 40 a day you need to move on a bit more speedily or this will take as long as a pregnancy!) Spermatogenesis takes 116 days, so you need to allow 116 days from the last cigarette until Happy Day for Super Sperm.

Other people have said it is easier to make a clean break and chuck away the packet and be done with it! I guess it depends upon the individual temperament and physiology! Also, perhaps how near you live to the shops! You can also put the money saved in a jar and watch it grow week by week!

For added motivation the following research has taken place:

Those who smoke run an added risk of fathering children who later develop cancer or leukaemia.

Cigarettes Per Day	Increased Risk
1-9	3%
10-20	31%
20+	42%

Based on Oxford Survey of Childhood Cancers. British Journal of Cancer.

See the following pages for a number of charts from relevant research studies.

For smoking father's babies there is over two and a half times the risk of malformation with 11 cigarettes a day or more. Slightly over double the number of malformed sperm with 31 or more cigarettes smoked per day.

Teeside Study
A very telling Research Study was conducted by Dr Barry Hemsworth of Teeside University. Male mice were given daily injections of nicotine. It was calculated according to body weight and blood volume that the amount of nicotine they were given equated to a fully-grown man smoking 20 cigarettes a day. Spermatogenesis in the mouse takes 11 days.

After 5 months of "moderate smoking" the first cohort of mice were mated. The female mice from these matings suffered a 16.4% in utero death rate, (roughly equivalent to human miscarriage). This works out at approximately one baby in six being lost. Of the remainder, 4.8% had suffered limb reduction deformities. **(21.2% major disaster rate).**

A second cohort were then allowed off their injections for a week, and then mated. As spermatogenesis in a mouse takes only 11 days, this was roughly the equivalent of a "one-third contaminated" sperm population, compared with the previous group.

The resultant matings produced a 13.1% in utero death-rate, and a 1.6% limb reduction deformity rate (exactly one-third the number of babies with malformed limbs). **(A 14.7% major disaster rate.)** A considerable improvement, although some nicotine was still present.

The final cohort was mated after 3 weeks entirely free from nicotine and the mother then suffered only 3.8% in utero losses, and there were no malformed limbs. **(Only a 3.8% disaster rate.)**

To show this more graphically

RESORBED/MISCARRIED

NICOTINE +	16.4%
NICOTINE 1/2	13.1%
NICOTINE -	3.8%

MALFORMED
(LIMB REDUCTION DEFORMITY, OR MISSING LIMBS)

NICOTINE +	4.8%
NICOTINE 1/2	1.6%
NICOTINE -	0%

This study is interesting for two reasons: It demonstrates that although a reduction in nicotine smoking does give some help, it is not enough. The whole process of spermatogenesis needs to take place free from this noxious element completely.

It poses the question, what could be achieved nationwide by healthy fatherhood?

Currently, 1 baby in 4 (25%) of all babies in the UK are miscarried. If those born alive are 700,000 (approximate figures), then in the region of 23,333 babies perish in the womb every year. How many of these family tragedies are down to a non-viable sperm?

Over 5,000 babies are born every year with limb reduction deformity. (1 child in 140 or 0.7%) How much of this could be prevented by no parent smoking?

At the very least, this should all be considered urgent for further research.

However, to obtain this research, a lot of pressure will have to be brought to bear by the general public, as the wealth, and therefore the influence, of the alcohol and tobacco firms, is immense. This is where you can help. See Final Chapter. Ask for what you want. Go on asking until you get it!

HAVOC CREATED BY TOBACCO

Tobacco in either parent increases risk of:

- Low Sperm Count
- Anovulation
- Miscarriage
- Premature Birth
- Malformation
- Hyperactivity
- Asthma
- Cot Death
- Learning Difficulties

Levels of Lead and Cadmium are increased, and levels of Selenium and Zinc are decreased.

Smoking - male - linked with:

- Decreased sperm density
- Less motile sperm
- Decreased sperm count
- Reduced testosterone secretion
- Powerful anti-vitamin C effect

Tobacco smoke contains more than 4,000 compounds, including: carbon monoxide, oxide of nitrogen, ammonia, aromatic hydrocarbons, hydrogen cyanide, vinyl chloride and nicotine.

Nicotine:

- Changes adrenaline and cortisol levels in the blood
- Causes foetal heart rate changes
- Decreases interplacental blood flow
- Effects placental amino acid uptake (foetal growth retardation)

Carbon monoxide:

- High carbon monoxide effects foetal blood flow to brain, heart and adrenal glands
- Effects brain and protein synthesis

Polycyclic aromatic hydrocarbons:
- Widely distributed mutagens and carcinogens
- Interferes with placental hormone activity

Cyanide:
- Contributes to retarded infant growth
- Decreases concentration of vitamin B12

HAVOC CREATED BY ALCOHOL

Alcohol increases risk of -
- Low sperm count
- Damaged sperm
- Poor motility
- Foetal alcohol syndrome
- Small baby
- Failure to thrive
- Deformed face and joints
- Hyperactivity
- Mental retardation

Alcohol - important factor in male reproductive failure - testicular toxin. Causes:
- Atrophy of semeniferous tubules
- Loss of sperm
- Increase in abnormal sperm
- Accumulation of female hormones
- Release of prolactin (a female hormone)

Alcohol induced zinc depletion is well-documented.
- Positive correlation with reduced zinc status and low birth weight and fetal malformations.
- Folic acid deficiency which results from alcohol-induced increased urinary excretion has been linked directly with the occurrence of spina bifida.
- Both ova and sperm are vulnerable to damage from drugs and chemicals before conception
- Ovum for 100 days prior to ovulation
- Sperm for 116 days before maturation

Pre-conception care should therefore start at least 4 months prior to conception to ensure perfect sperm and ova.

Street Drugs

Marijuana, Pot, Cannabis, Hash, Grass, Weed

- 4 times more dangerous than cigarette smoking

- 3 times more tar in the lungs and 5 times more carbon monoxide

Psychoactive substance to tetrahydrocannabinol (thc) - steroid structure found in the sex hormones and in certain hormones of the adrenal glands. This accumulates in the ovaries and testes.

Cannabis is by far the most chemically complex of illegal drugs. When smoked, the 421 component chemicals are combusted into over 2,000 chemicals. Some cause cancer. Others distribute themselves around the body and are deposited in fat-storage depots such as the testicles, the ovaries, the brain, the adrenals, the liver and other major organs. They remain in the cushions of fat surrounding the organs such as the heart and the kidneys, and slowly leak out producing unpredictable effects on body function. *Dr Garbial Nabas* has said

> *"Marijuana's impairing cellular effects on DNA can result in incomplete genetic information being transmitted to the offspring. This does not mean the babies of pot-smokers will have obvious birth defects. However, there is great danger that there will be subtle changes in physical or psychological characteristics, which may not be detected until much later in life. Therefore, the marijuana smoker may be playing Russian Roulette with unborn generations".*

He went on to explain that the user would also be at risk to other damaging effects of the drugs - on the brain, the lungs, the sex organs, and the immune system.

- Women - upsets menstrual cycle, tolerated and then restored.

- Men - lowers blood testosterone, lowers sperm count, greater than usual impotency and diminished libido. Sperm motility affected and an increase in number of abnormal sperm.

Affects the synthesis of DNA. In animals, linked with increased fetal deaths and malformations. *NB: Hair analysis done by Foresight often reveals very high levels of toxic metals following use of cannabis.*

At a Marijuana Workshop in 2002, *Mary Brett* recorded that cannabis psychosis could involve a complete mental breakdown including anxiety, depression, apathy, "dropping out", and paranoia. It was noted that the user became inflexible, hostile, lonely, miserable and remained childish and dependent. There is also a propensity to violence.

Cannabis users are more prone to lung cancer, rare head and neck cancers, chronic bronchitis and impaired immunity, this latter making them more vulnerable to all other diseases. There is also a five fold greater risk of heart attack.

Regarding reproduction, sperm production is decreased, and impotence is more likely.

Babies born to cannabis users are smaller, hyperactive, have behavioural and learning problems and are 10 times more likely to develop one form of leukaemia.

Effects on DNA have also been researched. The production of new cells in the body, white blood cells, sperm and foetal cells all involve the copying of the DNA which makes up our chromosomes. The active substance in cannabis THC (or Tetrahydrocannabinol) interferes with this process. This accelerates the death of the cell - which is called apoptosis. *A much fuller version of these articles can be seen on the* FORESIGHT *website.*

It is not hard to see how the psychosis induced by smoking "the weed" can lead to the doctors' prescribing "tranquillisers" to counteract the paranoia, anxiety, suicidal tendencies, violence and so on.

Thus, the slippery slopes get steeper, and the poor babies born subsequently more and more at risk to an ever-growing catalogue of disaster.

The roots of so-called "mental illness" become clearer all the time. It is not hard to see that poor food, and even quite mild involvement of smoking/drinking, or minimal use of "recreational drugs", coupled with the cerebral assault of copper and lead laden water and air, hidden allergies / infections / miasms and so on in the parents could induce some level of addiction in future generations. This might have remained with caffeinated drinks, a packet of fags, and the pint of beer, had the advent of designer drugs and pharmaceutical "solutions" not have arrived on the scene . . .

Fortunately, in almost all cases, preconceptual care can act as a firebreak. By giving the adults the expertise they need to recover - they have a chance to undo the damage, and give the baby a level playing field.

I think that only due to this can we stem this headlong rush into disaster with brain damage in-utero becoming the norm, so that each generation has more and more severe health and educational problems than the one before. This leading to an escalation in addiction, then drug wars, organised crime and ultimately a complete breakdown in society.

The salvation lies in a hard slog back to sanity using all the armoury of complimentary medicine to the full.

Cocaine and Crack
- In mice - teratogenic even at non-toxic levels for adult mice.

- Humans - decrease in weight of foetus, higher malformation rate and increased still-birth rate.

- Crack is a cocaine derivative which is purer than cocaine. Withdrawal symptoms in the new born are severe.

Heroin
Heroin and other opiate narcotics such as opium, morphine and codeine are all extremely addictive.

Decreased fertility and atrophy of the male accessory sex organs, decreased testosterone.
- 3 times more stillbirths

- 4 times more premature births

- 6 times more growth problems

Babies are born addicted to the drug and have to endure withdrawal. So parents have to endure the screaming which can last throughout babyhood, leading to childhood hyperactivity.

Medical Drugs

Anti-convulsants
Induce biochemical evidence of folate deficiency if the diet contains a barely adequate amount of this vitamin. This can result in malformations in the baby.

Antidepressants
Monoaminase blockers decrease sperm count and motility. Babies are born with central nervous system anomalies. Tricyclic antidepressants do not have the same effect.

Aspirin
When used in the first half of pregnancy, aspirin has been linked to lower subsequent IQ and lower ability to concentrate.

Tranquillisers and Sleeping Pills
Benzodiazepines taken during pregnancy have been linked to visible malformations, functional deficits and behavioural problems in babies. Studies show that mothers who take them during the first three months of pregnancy are 3.3 times more likely to have a baby with an oral cleft.

Betablockers
Phelezine, a betablocker, decreases sperm count and motility.

CHAPTER 5

GENITO-URINARY INFECTIONS

The most relevant bugs in the infertility scene are those that used to be known in times past as "Venereal Disease". They later became known as sexually transmitted diseases, or STDs. This also seemed a little too explicit in the present climate, so the Powers-That-Be have decided it is more politically correct to call them Genito-Urinary Infections, or GUIs. Therefore, the relevant hospital department is known as the "Genito-Urinary Medicine Department" which was abbreviated to the G.U.M. Clinic, and later called "The GUM Clinic", (which we might be forgiven for thinking was something to do with dentistry!) But this is where you go if you need to seek help. They need to see both of you. Ring your local large hospital for an appointment.

You do not need a letter from your GP to make an appointment at a GUM Clinic on the NHS. The range of infections routinely investigated in the GUM Clinics varies surprisingly. Some seem to have become rather stuck in a groove and only tackle Syphilis, Gonorrhoea, AIDS and Chlamydia. Others are quite with the modern scene and are screening for a wide range of infections as a matter of course. There are said to be 34 known conditions. More may turn up in the future.

A count up at one FORESIGHT clinic done in the 1990s, showed that 47% of males and 51 % of females coming for preconceptual care had a Genito-Urinary Infection.

Results of Infection Screen of 32 Men enrolled in the FORESIGHT Programme

69% tested low for sperm count and sperm activity

47% tested positive for one or more infections

100% of those with the following infections (8 cases) also exhibited low sperm count and low sperm activity:

Enterococcus
Staph aureus
Candida
E Coli
Strep milleri
Anaerobic bacteria

50-60% of those with the following infections (7 cases) also exhibited low sperm count and low sperm activity:

Ureaplasma
Haem Influenza

13 other cases exhibited low sperm count with no infection

Source: Report on Genitourinary Infection Screening of FORESIGHT Patients for a FORESIGHT Clinic (unpublished paper).

For the sake of ensuring anonymity we are not giving any further details.

Results of Infection Screen of 77 Women enrolled in the FORESIGHT Programme

49% had past history of infertility for 1 year or more

34% had past history of spontaneous abortion

51 % tested positive for one or more infections (cervical swab)

29% tested positive for Chlamydia (antibody levels)

Source: Report on Genitourinary Infection Screening of FORESIGHT Patients (unpublished paper).

Past Reproductive Problem	Infection Diagnosed by FORESIGHT (77 women tested)	Percentage of Diagnosed Infection Associated with Reproductive Problem
Spontaneous Abortion	B strep	46%
	Ureaplasma	27%
	Anaerobic bacteria	44%
	Candida	40%
	Gardnerella (BV)	16%
Infertility	B. strep	15%
	Ureaplasma	67%
	Anaerobic bacteria	38%
	Candida	50%
	Gardnerella (BV)	66%
Stillbirth	Anaerobic bacteria	6%
	Gardnerella (BV)	16%
Ectopic pregnancy	Mycoplasma (only 1 case)	100%

Another clinic in London found 29% of males (although 81 % of females) had an infection. Genito-urinary infection is unlikely to be the only problem preventing fertility, but dealing with it certainly contributes to the ability to have a baby, and also to the health of the future baby. Infection in the woman will make implantation less likely and, once a pregnancy is under way, will make miscarriage more likely. This can be a really heart-breaking situation where a baby has been waited for and wanted so desperately for a long time.

If the baby of the infected mother survives the first few months of pregnancy, and stays the course long enough for a live birth to take place, although probably premature, it is likely to be small for dates, because many nutrients and much maternal energy will have been channelled into fighting the infection. Zinc, in particular, is a nutrient that is both used by the body to power the immune system (thereby becoming much depleted in infection) and is also much needed by the future baby to effect his/her growth and development.

If the man has an infection he will give this to the woman, even if, at the time of conception, the woman appeared to be clear of it. *This is why it is always necessary for both partners to be tested and treated simultaneously.*

The Genito-Urinary Infections appear to stay around once they are caught. They are not fought off as easily as a cold or flu. The acute phase may be a short time of feeling rather as though you were struck down by the flu. At the time this may be perceived as a usual type of virus or lurgi or some sort. It may be shrugged off as the acute phase dies down. This does not mean, however, that the infection is over. It can linger in the woman's body, and, with the extra estrogens produced at the start of a pregnancy, the bugs can suddenly proliferate, and this may, sadly, end the pregnancy. It can linger in the man's body and will attack the sperm, and may ultimately destroy the sperm beds.

In other cases, localised irritation, frequency of urine sometimes with low back pain, may be present in either partner, and, in the woman, some discharge or vaginal irritation may persist. Pain on intercourse and acutely painful periods, also pain at the time of ovulation may start so insidiously and become so usual that many women accept this as "women's troubles".

I am often told by women that they have taken a collection of these vague (or not so vague) but distressing symptoms to their doctor. They have been dismissed with the "*most women have these sort of problems from time to time*" type of "reassurance". This is, of course, *true*! The FORESIGHT GUM Study showed that out of 55 women who had Genito-Urinary Infection, *none* had been diagnosed and treated by their GP. So, presumably many women *do* have these symptoms!

The most propitious course of action is for both partners to make a bee line for their local GUM Clinic, which is likely to be at the nearest large hospital. There the problems will be understood and coped with expertly. A referral is not necessary. I would advise a genito-urinary check up in all cases of infertility.

All that is necessary is to ring your nearest large hospital and ask if they have a "GUM Clinic". If they do not, they will certainly be able to tell you where the nearest one is. When you speak to the Clinic, ask if they cover the following:

Chlamydia	B Streptococcus
Gardnerella	Haemolytic Streptococcus
Ureaplasma	Streptococcus Millerii
Enterococcus	Mycoplasma
Eshericum Coli	Haemolytic Influenza
Anaerobic bacteria	Staphylococcus Aureas
Klebsiella	Candida
Herpes	

Some Clinics do not have a sufficiently powerful microscope to be able to scan for Ureaplasmas or Mycoplasmas. If you cannot get the latter two done on the NHS locally, it will be possible to get them done privately. FORESIGHT can advise you on request. Please send an SAE for information.

Both partners should attend, as otherwise the bugs can be passed to and fro, and the infection will keep recurring. The GUM Clinics appear to vary with what they do in the way of treatment. Some prescribe an antibiotic on the spot, and some report back to the couple's own GP. Some will be willing to report back to a nutritionist or homeopath, if this is who referred the couple, as they are seeing them about all their health problems.

Treatment from the GUM Clinic or your GP can be antibiotics. If these are used, they should be taken in conjunction with B-complex vitamins, and live yoghurt, also acidophilus and biodophilus to help the flora of both small and great intestine. Antibiotics tend to destroy friendly (necessary) bugs, as well as unfriendly ones.

If people would rather try an alternative to antibiotics any homeopath will be willing to make up a remedy called a "nosode" to counteract the relevant bug, or do a "whole person" approach with the relevant homeopathic remedies. Many herbalists are also very knowledgeable in this area. See Appendix V for how to find a homeopath or herbalist in your area.

In addition to antibiotics or homeopathic treatment, with the wife, the topical application of live yoghurt is also often found helpful. Douching with warm water and bicarbonate of soda is also recommended to counteract "hostile mucus", and it would seem likely that the "hostility" may sometimes be something to do with bugs present, although heavy levels of lead and mercury can also cause this, (more anon).

Health will also be reinforced by adding a few drops of tea-tree oil to the bath water. This will be obtainable from your local health store.

Other complementary and harmless aids which may assist the process (used in conjunction with antibiotics or nosodes) are said to be drinking Cranberry juice - now available in all the supermarkets - and taking a preparation made from grapefruit pips called "Citracidal" available in Health Stores.

Whatever method you favour, both of you need to return to the GUM Clinic a few weeks later to be checked out again, to see that, whatever therapy you decided upon, it did actually achieve the desired result. This is the only way to find out, as a lot of GUI are extremely hard to detect, many having almost no symptoms at all. There is usually no temperature rise.

Sometimes there is vaginal irritation, pain on intercourse etc, and sometimes not. In the male there may be frequency of urine or some local irritation. Often there are virtually no symptoms at all! In cases of infertility, it is always worth checking out, however, as this is the only certain way to discover if this is a factor impairing your fertility. We found 9 out of 15 infertile men in the Hertfordshire survey were positive, ie 60% of them had a bug on board *and that they were completely unaware of it.*

If the infection is chlamydia and it is not checked, it can continue in your wife during the pregnancy. The effects on the baby can be dire - if it survives the pregnancy, it may suffer from Chlamydial pneumonia (bugs in the lungs), which can later lead to asthma, as the surface of the lungs can be damaged.

Chlamydia can also lead to the baby suffering attacks of Otitis Media (middle ear infection - earache). An American study examined the exudate from the ears of a series of children with recurrent otitis media, and found that more than half of them were suffering from chlamydia in the middle ear.

Other studies have identified chlamydia as a source of gastro-enteritis, which can result in prolonged illness, even death. It is also well known for attacking the eyes of the newborn. Usually, this is detected and treated at birth, but occasionally the damage has been done and it can lead to impaired sight which is lifelong.

It is likely it can lie behind urinary tract infection in the child also.

It is therefore imperative that it is coped with effectively. The responsibility will be yours to follow up and make certain. The treatments do not always work first time, although most do. However, if you check and recheck as necessary, you will achieve after a few weeks, and this will lead to much improvement in your general health, and of course your fertility. Nothing but benefit all round. *Let's get cracking!*

Chlamydial Infections in Infants

50-70% of infants born to infected mothers.

Inclusion Conjunctivitis:
>35-50%
>chlamydial ocular infection
>neovascularization (pannus)
>conjunctival scarring

Pneumonitis:
>chronic pulmonary infiltrates
>afebrile course
>chronic respiratory sequelae

Otitis Media
>acute otitis media
>recurring illness

Gastro-enteritis
>can lead to serious illness

Unspecified viral disease
>may include urinary tract infection

Also: rhinitis, naso-pharyngitis, proctitis, vulvitis, failure to thrive.

Chlamydial Infection in Males

>30-50% of cases
>epididymitis
>non-gonococcal urethritis

University of Tampere in Finland
>Chlamydia found in the semen of
>>51.1 % of infertile men
>>23.2% of fertile men.

It was also noted the chlamydia was a common cause of prostitis.

Complications seen with other Major Infections and Possible Consequences

Group B-streptococci
    can cause amnionitis
    premature rupture of the membranes
    premature birth
    neonatal sepsis

Cytomegalovirus
    can cause blindness
    deafness
    acute microcephaly
    mental retardation
    cerebral palsy
    death

In the UK 2,800 infants are infected by Cytomegalovirus every year
500 a year suffer brain damage.

Herpes virus
    severe damage to the central nervous system, eyes, skin, liver.

Mycoplasma hominis
    53% of pregnant women lose the pregnancy.

Ureaplasma urealyticum
    up to 93% incidence of miscarriage, prematurity, neonatal
    morbidity, mortality

Other sexually transmitted infections
    infertility
    miscarriage
    prenatal damage.

Found in FORESIGHT Couples: 1995-98

(none of whom had been previously diagnosed or had suspected they had any infection.)

Chlamydia	B. Streptococcus
Gardnerella	Haemolytic Streptococcus
Ureaplasma	Streptococcus Millerii
Enterococcus	Mycoplasma
Eshericum Coli	Haemolytic Influenza
Anaerobic bacteria	Staphylococcus Aureas
Klebsiella	Candida

We would also advise testing for: Herpes, Gonorrhoea, AIDS and Papilloma virus. Also, while a blood sample is available and where medical personnel are willing: Cytomegalovirus Toxoplasmosis and Rubella, as these can lead to blindness, deafness, epilepsy and retardation in the infant. You need to ask if this can be arranged in advance as it will be in co-operation with another department in the hospital.

More Comprehensive Study - UK -109 FORESIGHT Patients - Men (more detailed analysis)

Total men tested	32
Total men tested with low sperm count activity	22
Total men tested with normal sperm count	7
Total men tested with sperm count not known	3
Total with infection	15
Low sperm count with infection	9
Low sperm count with no infection	13
Normal sperm count with infection	6
Normal sperm count with no infection	1

Infections seen with low sperm count:

Ureaplasma	3
Enterococcus	1
Staph Aureus	1
Candida	1
Haem Influenza	1
E Coli	3
Anaerobic Bacteria	1
Strep Millerii	1

NB: 9 men - 12 infections. Some had more than one infection.

Infections seen in men with normal sperm count, or count not known (but conception illusive):

B Strep	3
Chlamydia	1
Ureaplasma	2
Haem Influenza	1
Klebsiella	1

NB: 6 men - 8 infections.

CHAPTER 6

ALLERGY, REACTIVE HYPOGLYCAEMIA AND INTESTINAL INFESTATION

Allergic illness, reactive hypoglycaemia and intestinal parasites are three troublesome health "downers".

All or none of them may be relevant to you, and none may be directly relevant to the fertility question. However, anything that zaps the energy, overuses the available nutrients and/or makes for reliance on medicaments is unlikely to be entirely innocent.

I would examine the situation, and see if any of the following is useful to you.

"Allergy" is a term that is loosely used for any idiosyncratic and unpleasant reaction to a substance that is usually harmless. True allergy involves a breakdown of the immune system, and the medicine men can pinpoint this in various ways - by skin-prick tests, by giving drops under the tongue, by examining cells under a microscope and so on. Some substances are then identified as "true" allergies, while other adverse reactions are classified as "hyper-sensitivity" or "intolerance".

Be all that as it may, it is undeniable that many people find that a wide variety of afflictions will respond to the removal of a "trigger factor" from the environment. This includes eczema and other skin conditions, asthma, migraine, insomnia, depression, rhinitis (runny nose), diarrhoea, even cystitis and some times epilepsy.

Most often the offending substance is a commonly used food such as wheat, sugar and/or milk or, less commonly, any other foods. However, it can be something that is inhaled, such as leaking gas, pollen, hydro-carbons from traffic effluent, animal dandruff, house dust mite excreta, perfumes, and/or pungent smells that arise from household cleaning materials, to name but a few.

Reasons For Increased Incidence

People speculate on the reasons for the increase in allergy/intolerance/ sensitivity over the past few decades. As with all things that are part of real life, (as against taking place under tightly controlled laboratory conditions), it is probably bits of this and that, woven together and not separable into very coherent parts.

One thing I am sure it is not is the ubiquitous excuse called "STRESS". During the war years, the phenomenon of "allergy" was virtually unknown when fathers, husbands and sons were being killed in foreign lands, and when people were being bombed, overworked, made homeless, children separated from parents by evacuations and so on. Twenty years later, allergy was commonplace (manifesting as eczema, asthma, migraine, depression etc and sometimes insomnia, arthritis and epilepsy), although it took about a further couple of decades for all the different manifestations to be recognised.

Some of the more plausible explanations for the ever increasing numbers of sufferers are as follows:

- The decline of breast-feeding leading to early introduction of unsuitable and allergenic substitutes such as cow's milk formula with sugar (possibly laced with "Miltons" from sterilizing) and then on to "solid" food before the infant gut is ready to cope with the onslaught.

- The pollution of air with lead up until 1997 from traffic effluent as well as from scraping down old paintwork, and factory effluent, and occasionally from tap-water. The contamination of water with heavy metals and excess copper.

- The spraying of crops with chemicals such as pesticides, and the excess of nitrates (also moth-proofing and fire-proofing of soft furnishings and bedding) and the heavy use of chlorine in drinking water. All may lower the resistance to allergens by "downing" the immune system and preventing the gut flora from developing. All overuse zinc and other needed nutrients as the body struggles to eliminate the invaders.

- The widespread use of antibiotics with young children - mainly in response to otitis media - (which may be chlamydial in origin).

Antibiotics will play havoc with the intestinal bacteria needed for the proper breakdown of the food, and tend to induce over-growth of candida albicans in the gut. This can impair digestive processes and can crowd out other useful gut flora.

• The lack of trace minerals such as zinc, selenium and manganese, which act as cofactors with numerous enzyme systems. The cofactor is like the outboard motor on a dinghy, it provides the "Go-Factor"! This paucity is partly due to the poor quality of food. This means that enzymes necessary for the metabolism of the food may not be functioning. Paucity of these minerals, and of B complex vitamins is largely due to heavy consumption of refined carbohydrates.

• Foods grown with Sodium-Potassium-Phosphate fertiliser will be short of essential trace minerals. This includes almost all food that is not grown organically.

• Foods that are mass-produced in ways that are bound to affect the quality of the end product. Wheat, for example, is such a commercially important product that it has received much attention from "science". Efforts were made to find a way to breed a species that would produce extra grain to a stem. This was successful, but the plant was then top-heavy and so was easily blown over by the wind! A hormone was then dreamed up that prevented the stem from growing too tall. The short, heavy grains of wheat were then found to be too soft, and to be growing a grey fungus. A fungicide was then produced to kill the mould . . . Altogether I am told that wheat is now treated with 14 different chemicals before it is presented to us on the supermarket shelves. Residues of any or all of these may be present in the end product.

We could be forgiven for thinking that perhaps the white product is safer? Surely all this muck is sprayed onto the outside of the grain? However, studies have shown that the white flour is equally contaminated. (Husk and grain are ground together, before the "white dust" is sucked up and separated). The only solution is to eat organic bread, and cook with organic flour. Luckily these are now readily available in the supermarkets.

Some Foresight clinicians have found that many people who are sensitive to wheat and who exhibit a variety of symptoms after eating ordinary wheat products can nevertheless tolerate organically grown wheat. Dr Jean Monro, who is one of those foremost in the allergy field, has found about 2 out of 3 "wheat allergic" patients can eat the organically produced product. Wheat when grown inorganically is inevitably subjected to all these chemicals which may produce adverse reactions in sensitive people and, one can presume, in the foetus. However, organically grown wheat flour with the Soil Association label is to be found in most supermarkets.

- Milk is a very suspect product if not organically produced. Cows are no longer fed solely on grass, hay and leaf-feed. Some of their feed is grain, or "cow-cake", and this may not be organically grown.

They are not, so far as we know, (and I hope they never will be), being injected with the Monsanto-produced BST (extra estrogens). However, the practice has developed of milking cows while they are pregnant (to the detriment of cow and future calf) and this adds extra (natural) estrogens to the milk. This, despite the fact that it is widely known that we are all already in a state of hormonal imbalance with too many estrogens! These are a major cause of malformed (non-functional) sperm.

The milk is taken from the tubes of milking machines that have been cleaned down with Milton or a similar disinfectant. It is put into churns cleaned with another chemical. From the churns it is tipped into a tanker similarly sterilised.

How much extra female hormone and how much residue of these chemicals ends up in the milk we drink? On occasion, cows are treated with an organophosphate warble fly dressing. This will be absorbed into the bloodstream and thence will go into the milk. The cows react to their dressing with effects we would term "allergy" in the human population. How much warble fly dressing do we get? What does it do? Does it contribute to "cow's milk allergy"?

- Additives to food, that are intentional: tartrazine in particular, (otherwise known as E102), has been shown to lower zinc in the blood, and raise it in the urine. *(This may be because zinc coats the particles of tartrazine in order for them to be safely excreted by the kidney without inflicting damage on the way out?)* Whatever the mechanism, tartrazine squanders a lot of the body's zinc stores. Possibly for this reason, tartrazine causes eczema, asthma and hyperactivity in children. A huge variety of additives are in manufactured food. Many of these produce "allergic reactions" there and then. It is likely they also squander essential nutrients, as tartrazine does. These nutrients would have been the vital cofactors for the enzyme systems that would have facilitated the digestion of other foods. In this way, these artificial additives deliver a double whammy. *Zinc is an essential mineral for sperm integrity.*

- Other "additives" arrive in the foods by default rather than by design! Organophosphate pesticides tend to be used liberally on vegetables, fruit and grain unless these are specifically grown organically. By law, the pesticides must not be used less than 3 weeks before the date for harvesting. However, it is unlikely this embargo is rigidly adhered to, and even should this be so, there may not have been enough wind and rain in the interim to render the product pristine! In fact, tests by Friends of the Earth, have found illegal residues in more than half the foods they tested on more than one occasion. The latest count up in 2000 revealed 44% of foods they tested had residues.

(Organophosphate pesticides inhibit the action of the choline-containing enzymes. These enzymes are needed to carry manganese across the gut/blood barrier, so that manganese can circulate in the blood. In this way, the pesticides can cause manganese deficiency. Manganese is needed to carry oxygen to the mitochondria of the cell).

Zinc and manganese are two of the most essential elements for the proper assimilation of food. Without them the digestive system is a sinking ship! (They are also two of the most essential elements for fertility, and for foetal health!)

- Vaccinations. The ubiquitous jabs which lie behind so much controversy. First there is the active substance - designed to stimulate what must be an immature and already beleaguered immune system in a tiny baby. Then there is the cattle lymph that the substance is "floated" in. We know cow's milk, taken into the digestive tract, is often found to be allergenic. How allergenic is cattle lymph going directly into the circulatory system?

  How long does it take the body to flush it out if the blood completely, if it can, and does it do any damage on the way? What effect does it have on the baby's blood, liver, kidneys and brain, - when will this be studied? Does it affect the baby's ovary or testicle? *Ask your mother if you had a bad reaction to any of your jabs.*

- Hair dyes. They contain many suspect chemicals and are absorbed through the scalp and appear in the urine 30 minutes after application. They have been linked to bladder cancer.

- Fluoride. I hope you are not unlucky enough to have mass fluoridation foisted upon you via your drinking water. Fluoride is known to lower the immune system - amongst other things - so may contribute something to this crowded list.

All of these environmental hazards may have weakened your immune system and made you more vulnerable to food-related disorders. This may be the reason why you are allergic.

Is it likely you have an allergy?
Do you suffer form any skin complaint, breathing disorder, head pains, sleeplessness - or alternatively the tendency to fall asleep at awkward moments throughout the day - do you have flatulence, or a perpetually runny nose, a tendency to upset stomach, or diarrhoea, or do you need to urinate frequently?

If so, and especially if you are on repeat prescription medication for any of these misfortunes, this may be contributing to the infertility.

As we have discussed, wheat and milk are the two most likely candidates for examination. As a very broad generalisation - and therefore a fallible one - the wheat allergics tend to be thin, hyperactive, voluble, irritable, restless and quick tempered. They tend to have irritable skins, runny noses, diarrhoea, cystitis, joint pain, muscle pains and to find sleep elusive. The wheat allergics may react to all the gluten-grains - wheat, oats, barley and rye. This is known as coeliac condition.

The milk allergics tend more to be heavy, sleepy, headachy, tired all the time, possibly asthmatic, withdrawn, depressed and weary. They too can suffer joint pain, and skin problems.

If you suspect a gluten allergy, it is possible to test this out quite easily by leaving wheat, oats, barley and rye out of the diet altogether. However, when reintroduced, the allergy may be more marked and the grain may then produce bloating, stomach pains and quite violent diarrhoea. Choose a good day to experiment!

If you entirely withdraw all dairy products, it is not safe to reintroduce them except under medical supervision - at least inform your doctor that you are thinking of doing this, as the subsequent reintroduction can be dangerous, with serious allergic reactions even anaphylactic shock - stopping of the heart.

It may be better simply to lower the intake of cow products to a very small amount each day, as this may minimise the symptoms. Otherwise seek professional advice, preferably from a doctor or nutritionist experienced with allergy. If you do have a very bad reaction, try taking some bicarbonate of soda - a teaspoon in a glass of water to "turn it off".

Other allergies may be easier to spot and less troublesome to eliminate. Keep a food diary, and write down exactly what you eat each day, and make a note of any adverse reactions. After a month or so - yes, it might take that long - it should be possible to spot "cause and effect". The effects may be fairly immediate, or may not be for any time up to 4 days - although most will be sooner than that. This may make it all quite difficult, but a pattern will probably emerge.

If the DIY approach all gets a bit too complicated there are doctors who specialise in this field. Also from all the nutritional colleges there are trained nutritionists with a good understanding of food allergy. I will list these colleges among Useful Addresses in Appendix V or write directly to FORESIGHT - with an SAE - and ask us for whoever you need.

If you find your health is significantly improved on an adapted diet, you will find more useful addresses, a few basic recipes, and books in the relevant lists at the back.

FORESIGHT has a lending library, if you join us, you can borrow useful books. Ask the Resource Centre for the list.

Vera Walker's Study

A fascinating survey by Dr Vera Walker of the UK, once President of the British Allergists Association, demonstrates the link between dyslexia and other common illnesses in school-children and also how these problems tend to "run in families".

I will show her four tables of conditions present in her patients and the numbers among close relatives.

Table I
1,534 Migraine Families

Migraine	4,538
Asthma	1,058
Eczema or Urticaria	1,548
Dyslexia	210
Coeliac	103
Epilepsy	258
Schizophrenia	86
Other Mental Illness	540

Table II
138 Dyslexia Families

Dyslexia	256
Migraine	336
Asthma	128
Eczema or Urticaria	202
Coeliac	202
Epilepsy	31
Schizophrenia	18
Other Mental Illness	64

Table III
83 Coeliac Families

Coeliac	108
Migraine	265
Asthma	73
Eczema or Urticaria	117
Dyslexia	7
Epilepsy	16
Schizophrenia	5
Other Mental Illness	47

Table IV
84 Schizophrenia Families

Schizophrenia	91
Migraine	246
Asthma	83
Eczema or Urticaria	104
Dyslexia	25
Coeliac	22
Epilepsy	4
Other Mental Illness	61

Dr Vera Walker was a really splendid lady who was Founder and President of the British Association of Allergists, long before allergy was acceptable as a diagnosis, let alone popular. She gave me very valuable advice, information and moral support when I was first setting up FORESIGHT. We discussed how Allergy/Malabsorption/Nutrient Deficiency conditions ran in families, and she went through her patient's records to check this out. The overlap proved to be remarkable. Close relations include mother, father, siblings, son, daughter. She did not extend the net further, as it could have got too confusing and more chancy.

Hypoglycaemia

Reactive hypoglycaemia or swinging blood sugar is another modern food-related disorder. For whatever reason the pancreatic function is unstable and the control of the blood sugar levels is inadequate.

This condition may be due to a shortage of chromium, zinc, manganese, cobalt and selenium, the minerals which help the pancreas to stabilise the blood sugar, also the B-vitamin pantothenic acid. It is possible also that there may be built-in faults in the pancreas due to a shortage of one or more of these nutrients before birth.

The trigger can be a sudden high intake of alcohol, sugar, confectionery and caffeine-containing foods and drinks - coffee, chocolate, cola and to a lesser degree, tea.

The blood sugar will shoot up in response to the stimulus of any of these substances, and will give a feeling of elation and a rush of energy. As this is very uncontrolled, it will be short lived. It will be followed by a feeling of fatigue, possibly by falling asleep, but if this is not possible due to the circumstances, often by irritability, or even violent outbursts of temper. According to the basic temperament, the reaction may be exasperation, rage, impatience with your own or other's limitations, or despair and withdrawal.

The rise will be followed by the fall, as night follows day, and this can make the hypoglycaemic very bewildering to live with.

Alcohol, and possibly some new street drugs, give the highest lift and the furthest fall. White sugar, which is also naked calories, comes not far behind.

A cigarette can also cause a rise in blood sugar, and the medium to heavy smoker will experience the same yo-yoing of blood sugar and mood round the day.

The hypoglycaemic will often see the rise as the "normal" state of affairs, with himself very much at the apex of things and in total command, and will view the "low" as the state he is reduced to due to the "stress" induced by the inadequacies and incompetence of those around him!

Some hypoglycaemics can yo-yo their way up to positions of great power and glory, if the peaks manifest at some very propitious moments and the lows are kept concealed from the outside world - at least until some weary colleague or partner blows the gaff in an unexpurgated biography! However, most bumble along, in and out of the peaks and troughs, cushioned by stalwart family and colleagues who keep the situation within bounds as best they may.

The solution is two fold. Firstly, avoid alcohol, cigarettes, sugar, coffee, cola and tea, or keep the consumption of the last four down to a minimum. Use brown raw sugar and decaffeinated coffee whenever possible where consumption is inevitable.

Secondly, seek help with adjusting your levels of zinc, manganese, chromium, cobalt, selenium and B Complex vitamins.

The difference will astound you, but even more, those around you!

Intestinal Parasites
It seems that until comparatively recently, very little was known about intestinal parasites (bugs in the gut).

It now emerges that apart from threadworms and candida (which we have all known about for a long time), there are quite a number of other little creatures that can take up residence in the intestine and, by stealing a lot of the nutrients from our food as it passes through the body, can cause havoc with our general health.

It used to be thought that we had to travel to far outreaches of the planet to pick up these foreign fellows. Generally the suggestion that we might have them on board was not taken seriously by the very British

GP unless we could produce a history of some outlandish and exotic journeys.

Apparently this is now a thing of the past. We can get a wide variety of different parasites from the drinking water and/or quite homely food without journeying as far as the end of the road.

So, how do we guess if we may have them? The classic sign is a condition known as "irritable bowel syndrome" - bloating after meals, pain, diarrhoea, fatigue, general malaise, irritation of the anus and sometimes loss of weight, despite eating quite a lot. You may only have some of these symptoms.

For once, the diagnosis can be quite straightforward. Any qualified nutritionist can arrange a stool test, and some very stalwart and commendable people can examine it, and let us know in due course what we have and how to get rid of them!

If you have discomfort in this way - and have probably been told that it is all due to "stress" - it will be well worth the effort to get rid of it.

Two quite commonly found parasites are called giardia lamblia and blastocystic hominus. Again, as with the genito-urinary infections, they can be tackled via the GP, with antibiotics, followed up with B complex vitamins, acidophilus and so on, or you can consult a homeopath who can tackle this with nosodes. (Addresses in Appendix IV).

I would revisit your nutritionist and recheck with another stool sample a few weeks later to make sure the regime has "worked". Some parasites can be quite hard to eliminate, and can keep "returning". (The ones left behind increase in numbers again). As before, with the GUI, my motto would be "If in doubt, check it out". You have very little to lose - and such a lot to gain. Continue to pursue this with follow-up stool tests and treatment until you feel quite certain that your guts are as they should be - and until there is a clear stool test.

If your practitioner wants to know where to send stool samples, see Parascope among the Useful Addresses.

CHAPTER 7

MINERAL METABOLISM

From the outset, all of us involved with Foresight have found mineral metabolism of primary importance regarding fertility. Many of the doctors whose work was referred to in former chapters have demonstrated this in their research.

Our objective in doing hair analyses has been to optimise the mineral levels in the prospective mother and the father, that are known to be of vital importance to fertility, and later to optimum foetal development.

At the same time, we lower the levels of those heavy metals known to be toxic, which inhibit fertility and work to the detriment of sperm development and ultimately to the foetus.

All the research that has been done has confirmed, time and again, that these adjustments can make the difference between a happy ending and a tragic one to any pregnancy. This way we can make practical use of the knowledge produced by this research.

Lead and Other Toxic Metals
The evidence on lead and cadmium has been around for a long time.

Researchers such as *Phil Needleman, George Wibberley, Derek Bryce-Smith* and *Neil Ward* have produced many scientific papers, showing the disadvantages ranging from infertility, miscarriage and stillbirth to mental retardation, skeletal deformities and spina bifida. Also there were other health problems such as eczema, hyperactivity and learning difficulties, in babies where lead and cadmium levels have been significant but not high enough to cause deformity.

The following three charts are those of an autistic child aged 10.5 years, over two and a half years. Note the drop in toxic metals and rise of all the essential minerals, particularly zinc, manganese and selenium. These changes have seen huge clinical improvement in the child's condition.

CHART 1

Name: Master S.R. Date: August 1996

	Your Results	**Recommended Values**	
Calcium:	172.00	400.00	mg/kg
Magnesium:	31.70	35.00	mg/kg
Potassium:	69.10	75.00	mg/kg
Iron:	28.30	30.00	mg/kg
Chromium:	0.29	0.8	mg/kg
Cobalt:	0.14	0.25	mg/kg
Copper:	13.20	20.00	mg/kg
Manganese:	0.64	1.5	mg/kg
Nickel:	0.29	0.8	mg/kg
Selenium:	1.14	2.25	mg/kg
Zinc:	91.00	185.00	mg/kg

		Threshold Values	
Aluminium:	8.91	2.5	mg/kg
Cadmium:	0.11	0.25	mg/kg
Mercury:	0.02	0.4	mg/kg
Lead:	1.13	1.0	mg/kg
Molybdenum:	0.24	-	mg/kg
Vanadium:	0.19	-	mg/kg
Rubidium:	0.02	-	mg/kg
Sodium:	56.00	-	mg/kg

Note particularly low manganese, selenium and zinc and very high aluminium.

CHART 2

Name: Master S.R.   Date: January 1997

	Your Results	**Recommended Values**	
Calcium:	417.00	400.00	mg/kg
Magnesium:	35.20	35.00	mg/kg
Potassium:	76.40	75.00	mg/kg
Iron:	41.20	30.00	mg/kg
Chromium:	0.67	0.8	mg/kg
Cobalt:	0.22	0.25	mg/kg
Copper:	17.30	20.00	mg/kg
Manganese:	1.28	1.5	mg/kg
Nickel:	0.66	0.8	mg/kg
Selenium:	1.72	2.25	mg/kg
Zinc:	119.00	185.00	mg/kg

		Threshold Values	
Aluminium:	1.29	2.5	mg/kg
Cadmium:	0.03	0.25	mg/kg
Mercury:	0.04	0.4	mg/kg
Lead:	2.73	1.0	mg/kg
Molybdenum:	0.26	-	mg/kg
Vanadium:	0.18	-	mg/kg
Rubidium:	0.08	-	mg/kg
Sodium:	75.00	-	mg/kg

CHART 3

Name: Master S.R.   Date: March 1999

	Your Results	**Recommended Values**	
Calcium:	376.00	400.00	mg/kg
Magnesium:	36.4	35.00	mg/kg
Potassium:	44.3	75.00	mg/kg
Iron:	36.8	30.00	mg/kg
Chromium:	0.92	0.8	mg/kg
Cobalt:	0.22	0.25	mg/kg
Copper:	11.50	20.00	mg/kg
Manganese:	2.18	1.5	mg/kg
Nickel:	0.72	0.8	mg/kg
Selenium:	2.61	2.25	mg/kg
Zinc:	175.00	185.00	mg/kg

		Threshold Values	
Aluminium:	1.99	2.5	mg/kg
Cadmium:	0.15	0.25	mg/kg
Mercury:	0.04	0.4	mg/kg
Lead:	0.61	1.0	mg/kg
Molybdenum:	0.12	-	mg/kg
Vanadium:	0.17	-	mg/kg
Rubidium:		-	mg/kg
Sodium:	54.40	-	mg/kg

This is the text of a letter we received from the mother of the child approximately 9 months after the hair analysis on the previous page:

"It has been some time since S was rechecked and I thought you would be interested to know how he is doing.

He has been 'gluten free' now for nearly 3 years. The change in his behaviour, concentration, ability to learn has been remarkable. School life is very happy for S: everyday we get positive feedback from the teacher and language therapist. He is also enjoying horseriding, sailing, cycling, dance lessons and swimming. I suspect, though, that his levels will be disappointing. When we were first in touch with you (mid 1996) you mentioned a number of possibilities. Gluten and dairy were the obvious culprits and we have seen wonderful changes since eliminating these from his diet. However, this summer, S suffered constantly from diarrhoea. Despite three stool tests nothing was revealed as untoward. It was very frustrating. In your original letter you had mentioned the possibility of giardia, I read up about it, and after much effort, persuaded the GP to test for this. Sure enough, the bug was found and S has recently treated for giardia with metronidazole. It has been the only course of antibiotics for over three years, as we generally use homeopathic remedies. During the course of treatment we gave him lactobacillus acidophilus and caprilic acid. We are awaiting the results of a retest but undoubtedly this will have affected his levels.

Otherwise we are continuing the glutamine; borage oil and trace minerals, but hope we can start to get it right for him."

S.R. continues to improve.

The following two charts are that of a 6 year old child, who suffered from hyperactivity, irritability, diarrhoea, panic attacks and night sweats.

CHART 1

Name: J.K   Date: September 1996

	Your Results	**Recommended Values**	
Calcium:	137.00	400.00	mg/kg
Magnesium:	31.00	35.00	mg/kg
Potassium:	63.00	75.00	mg/kg
Iron:	31.00	30.00	mg/kg
Chromium:	0.44	0.8	mg/kg
Cobalt:	0.13	0.25	mg/kg
Copper:	16.00	20.00	mg/kg
Manganese:	0.39	1.5	mg/kg
Nickel:	0.48	0.8	mg/kg
Selenium:	1.09	2.25	mg/kg
Zinc:	123.00	185.00	mg/kg

		Threshold Values	
Aluminium:	1.02	2.5	mg/kg
Cadmium:	0.02	0.25	mg/kg
Mercury:	0.01	0.4	mg/kg
Lead:	1.03	1.0	mg/kg

Hyperactivity is usually low manganese and zinc. Irritability and diarrhoea can result from low zinc. Panic attacks and night sweats can be lack of magnesium. All may owe something to organophosphate pesticides.

CHART 2

Name: J.K.   Date: March 1997

	Your Results	**Recommended Values**	
Calcium:	468.00	400.00	mg/kg
Magnesium:	48.00	35.00	mg/kg
Potassium:	75.00	75.00	mg/kg
Iron:	50.00	30.00	mg/kg
Chromium:	1.46	0.8	mg/kg
Cobalt:	0.26	0.25	mg/kg
Copper:	23.00	20.00	mg/kg
Manganese:	1.96	1.5	mg/kg
Nickel:	0.99	0.8	mg/kg
Selenium:	2.99	2.25	mg/kg
Zinc:	189.00	185.00	mg/kg
		Threshold Values	
Aluminium:	1.12	2.5	mg/kg
Cadmium:	0.10	0.25	mg/kg
Mercury:	0.07	0.4	mg/kg
Lead:	1.52	1.0	mg/kg

The child's hyperactivity has subsided, he is less aggressive and the diarrhoea is less frequent.

These two charts are for a four year old boy - hyperactive and allergic illness; aggressive and poor concentration. Found to be allergic to tomatoes, white flour, dairy products, oranges and grapes.

CHART 1

Name: Master A.G.   Date: November 1995

	Your Results	Recommended Values	
Calcium:	318.00	400.00	mg/kg
Magnesium:	42.00	35.00	mg/kg
Potassium:	75.00	75.00	mg/kg
Iron:	31.00	30.00	mg/kg
Chromium:	1.02	0.8	mg/kg
Cobalt:	0.14	0.25	mg/kg
Copper:	15.00	20.00	mg/kg
Manganese:	1.18	1.5	mg/kg
Nickel:	0.44	0.8	mg/kg
Selenium:	1.32	2.25	mg/kg
Zinc:	94.00	185.00	mg/kg

		Threshold Values	
Aluminium:	1.02	2.5	mg/kg
Cadmium:	0.01	0.25	mg/kg
Mercury:	0.01	0.4	mg/kg
Lead:	0.72	1.0	mg/kg

CHART 2

Name: Master A.G.   Date: January 1999

	Your Results	**Recommended Values**	
Calcium:	398.00	400.00	mg/kg
Magnesium:	47.00	35.00	mg/kg
Potassium:	79.00	75.00	mg/kg
Iron:	42.00	30.00	mg/kg
Chromium:	1.72	0.8	mg/kg
Cobalt:	0.24	0.25	mg/kg
Copper:	24.10	20.00	mg/kg
Manganese:	1.74	1.5	mg/kg
Nickel:	1.39	0.8	mg/kg
Selenium:	2.43	2.25	mg/kg
Zinc:	178.00	185.00	mg/kg

		Threshold Values	
Aluminium:	1.14	2.5	mg/kg
Cadmium:	0.17	0.25	mg/kg
Mercury:	0.13	0.4	mg/kg
Lead:	1.47	1.0	mg/kg
Molybdenum:	0.14	-	mg/kg
Vanadium:	0.24	-	mg/kg
Rubidium:	0.11	-	mg/kg
Sodium:	74.00	-	mg/kg

Huge improvements over 3 years. *"In the past year A has gained a lot more control, is less impulsive, less aggressive. He smiles and laughs a lot more, has made friends in school and is generally easier to live with. He is in mainstream class at school and is now reading at age 7-8 years and is an average student. Still a bit of difficulty with letter formation."*

What all these children might have been spared - and their parents - by preconceptual mineral adjustment!

Interestingly, the research Foresight did at the University of Surrey in 1992, showed that tobacco increased the levels of cadmium in the hair, and decreased those of zinc and iron. Alcohol intake also decreased levels of zinc and iron.

Other work from the same study strongly linked male fertility to levels of cadmium (low) and levels of zinc (high) and more tenuously to levels of iron (high).

Hair Analysis to Detect Essential Trace Mineral Deficiencies and High Levels of Toxic Metals.

A Brief History
Hair analysis for the detection of aberrant mineral and metal levels has been the lynch-pin of Foresight's work since the 1970's. As mentioned previously, in the early 70's, Dr Elizabeth Lodge-Rees, pioneered this technique for her paediatric practice.

She wondered about the potential of this technique for assessing her child patients, especially those brought to her with learning difficulties and hyperactivity.

Now there are a number of laboratories all over the world providing hair analysis, and almost any requirement for mineral supplementation can be met.

There is now a Hair Analysis Standardisation Board, and the Association of Elemental Substance Testing Laboratories, and standardised powdered human hair samples are regularly used for quality control throughout the industry.

In his book written in 1983, Dr Jeff Bland told us

> *"The significant increase in appreciation of the role that these elements play in human health and disease has led health practitioners to demand better ways of assessing mineral status in their patients. Hair mineral testing provides itself as a potentially useful technique, in that hair is easy to obtain, store, transport, and relatively easy to analyse, thereby providing significant information about trace mineral status, both of the essential and the toxic mineral."*

In the intervening 17 years, this *"potentially useful technique"* has certainly proved its worth.

In the mid 70's, I was working closely with *Dr Lodge-Rees,* helping mothers of hyperactive children to send samples to her laboratory Mineralab in the United States.

In 1978, with a group of friends, I founded Foresight, and was joined by 7 doctors who were interested in diet, allergy and homeopathy. They also started using the mineral readings.

In 1985, *Dr Stephen Davies* founded Biolab in London, and things became much easier. Foresight used Biolab for a some years until the University of Surrey took over doing the analyses as part of a long research programme under Dr Neil Ward. After 9 years we outgrew the capacity of the facility at the University, and installed our own laboratory in premises in Hampshire.

Interpreting the data
There are a number of different typical patterns that we see, and in fact, most charts are a mixture of these, - nothing clear-cut! They reflect the very diverse life-styles, heredity and environment of the couples who come to us. Prospective parents as a group are something of a microcosm of the human race.

The Following Are Classic Patterns
Charts with all the essential minerals on the low side: this can reflect a poor diet, weight loss programmes, anorexia, a recent infection, or a malabsorption condition, possibly coeliac condition, cow's milk allergy,

candida albicans of the gut, an intestinal parasitic infestation or just low stomach acid. (This last improves with Vitamin E.)

Charts with low essential minerals, especially Calcium, Magnesium, Zinc, Selenium and Manganese, but quite high toxic metals: This may reflect a high level of pollution. This may cause the beneficial minerals to be squandered as they coat (chelate) the toxic metals to take them out of the body.

High Toxic Metals: this may often reflect the smoking and the alcohol intake. Smokers have a much higher level of cadmium and often of lead. This is understandable as tobacco is said to contain cadmium and lead. The raised levels in those who drink a significant amount of alcohol are harder to understand, but it is a consistent pattern. It may reflect inhibited liver and kidney functions, as these organs may be stressed by eliminating the alcohol. Cannabis also produces a less predictable but wide range of high toxic metals.

High **lead** is quite usual and is the result of tap water in old lead water pipes, newsprint and old lead paint which is powdering. Scraping down old paint work is an especially common cause of high lead.

High **cadmium** may be the result of cigarette smoke, and more rarely, burning rubber (such as tyre effluent at Brand's Hatch).

Mercury can come from dental amalgams, tuna fish and swordfish.

Aluminium comes from pots, pans, kettles, and other kitchen utensils and from tea bags, foil wrap, foil dishes of cook-chill foods, "Coffee-mate", antacids - read the labels - and from the linings of some salt containers and container-cartons. Some juice cartons are aluminium-lined. Cut them open and have a look!

Selenium will also be lower in the smoker as the lungs use selenium to protect cells from damage. It is also lower in asthma patients. Both groups benefit from supplementation.

Chromium and **cobalt** are usually seen to be lower where there is significant use of alcohol, or overuse of sugar and refined carbohydrates.

The absorption of **manganese** will be inhibited by the dysfunction of the choline-containing enzymes in the presence of organophosphate pesticides. We have observed the low manganese in people working with organophosphate pesticides such as in nurseries and greenhouses, owning pets who wear flea collars or are treated with anti-flea drops on the neck, having new (moth-proofed) furnishings and so on.

Zinc will be chased down by stress, unhappiness, infection, injury or surgery. Also by high levels of copper or lead from the tap water, and by commonly used "fertility" drugs in the women. Also, alcohol and smoking will lower levels as demonstrated in the charts.

Most modern food is depleted of essential nutrients by methods of production and by processing, so quite large deficiencies are very common.

In practice, the only essential mineral that is quite often shown to rise too high is **copper**. Copper can be raised by exogenous hormones, copper water pipes and tanks, and some copper-containing algaecides in swimming pools. It is also present in hair dyes that contain henna. This latter can contaminate the sample.

Nickel is needed for healthy heart, liver and kidney function. Nickel may go down if the kidneys are stressed by infection.

Sodium and **potassium** can both be elevated in the presence of a liver problem, kidney infection or a high level of toxic metal.

Everybody's chart is different, but most people have a mixture of patterns. Some minerals work together and the presence of one will enhance the absorption and utilisation of another, iron=copper, zinc=manganese, calcium=magnesium. Others are antagonistic and will compete for the "binding sites" in the intestine from where they will be absorbed. Synergistic minerals can sometimes cause a lack of their counterpart by overusing the pathways, ie if you give calcium, the magnesium level will drop, or vice-versa. You must therefore always compensate when you supplement either.

The more that is known about the lifestyle and problems the more interesting it is reading charts. If we search enough, the reason for aberrant levels will be revealed in the person's environment, or previous environment, as high levels - good or bad - can often persist for some time.

Here are some charts of men who had fertility problems, showing what we did, and who was born afterwards!

The following chart is that of a 42 year old man who suffered from infertility. Lead went down, and zinc (among other things) went up. He later had a daughter.

CHART 1

Name: Mr J.P.   Date: November 1996

	Your Results	Recommended Values	
Calcium:	556.40	400.00	mg/kg
Magnesium:	47.30	35.00	mg/kg
Potassium:	84.60	75.00	mg/kg
Iron:	44.60	30.00	mg/kg
Chromium:	1.23	0.8	mg/kg
Cobalt:	0.24	0.25	mg/kg
Copper:	23.80	20.00	mg/kg
Manganese:	1.66	1.5	mg/kg
Nickel:	1.20	0.8	mg/kg
Selenium:	2.66	2.25	mg/kg
Zinc:	166.80	185.00	mg/kg

		Threshold Values	
Aluminium:	1.23	2.5	mg/kg
Cadmium:	0.12	0.25	mg/kg
Mercury:	0.16	0.4	mg/kg
Lead:	3.01	1.0	mg/kg
Molybdenum:	0.23	0.18	mg/kg
Vanadium:	0.30	0.18	mg/kg
Rubidium:	0.16	-	mg/kg
Sodium:	67.00	94.00	mg/kg

CHART 2

Name: Mr J.P.   Date: May 1997

	Your Results	**Recommended Values**	
Calcium:	560.90	400.00	mg/kg
Magnesium:	51.00	35.00	mg/kg
Potassium:	79.80	75.00	mg/kg
Iron:	43.90	30.00	mg/kg
Chromium:	1.36	0.8	mg/kg
Cobalt:	0.24	0.25	mg/kg
Copper:	22.90	20.00	mg/kg
Manganese:	2.16	1.5	mg/kg
Nickel:	1.13	0.8	mg/kg
Selenium:	2.93	2.25	mg/kg
Zinc:	183.70	185.00	mg/kg
		Threshold Values	
Aluminium:	1.13	2.5	mg/kg
Cadmium:	0.11	0.25	mg/kg
Mercury:	0.13	0.4	mg/kg
Lead:	1.96	1.0	mg/kg
Molybdenum:	0.27	0.18	mg/kg
Vanadium:	0.29	0.18	mg/kg
Rubidium:	0.20	-	mg/kg
Sodium:	79.00	94.00	mg/kg

Zinc level rose, lead level fell and they had a daughter.

The following two charts are for a 36 year old man who had suffered from infertility. After the programme, he had a daughter.

CHART 1

Name:	Mr J.A		Date: March 1996	
		Your Results	**Recommended Values**	
Calcium:		547.00	400.00	mg/kg
Magnesium:		60.00	35.00	mg/kg
Potassium:		109.00	75.00	mg/kg
Iron:		47.00	30.00	mg/kg
Chromium:		0.89	0.8	mg/kg
Cobalt:		0.17	0.25	mg/kg
Copper:		22.00	20.00	mg/kg
Manganese:		1.33	1.5	mg/kg
Nickel:		1.45	0.8	mg/kg
Selenium:		2.74	2.25	mg/kg
Zinc:		161.00	185.00	mg/kg
			Threshold Values	
Aluminium:		1.89	2.5	mg/kg
Cadmium:		0.09	0.25	mg/kg
Mercury:		0.12	0.4	mg/kg
Lead:		2.10	1.0	mg/kg

CHART 2

Name: Mr J.A.   Date: September 1997

	Your Results	**Recommended Values**	
Calcium:	579.00	400.00	mg/kg
Magnesium:	59.00	35.00	mg/kg
Potassium:	98.00	75.00	mg/kg
Iron:	47.00	30.00	mg/kg
Chromium:	1.27	0.8	mg/kg
Cobalt:	0.26	0.25	mg/kg
Copper:	22.00	20.00	mg/kg
Manganese:	1.94	1.5	mg/kg
Nickel:	1.29	0.8	mg/kg
Selenium:	3.01	2.25	mg/kg
Zinc:	173.00	185.00	mg/kg
		Threshold Values	
Aluminium:	1.46	2.5	mg/kg
Cadmium:	0.09	0.25	mg/kg
Mercury:	0.13	0.4	mg/kg
Lead:	1.44	1.0	mg/kg

Lead went down, cobalt, (B12) manganese and zinc levels rose and they had a daughter.

These two charts are for a 36 year old man who had suffered from infertility. After the programme he fathered twins!

CHART 1

Name: Mr J.B.   Date: February 1997

	Your Results	Recommended Values	
Calcium:	424.00	400.00	mg/kg
Magnesium:	45.00	35.00	mg/kg
Potassium:	90.00	75.00	mg/kg
Iron:	47.00	30.00	mg/kg
Chromium:	1.98	0.8	mg/kg
Cobalt:	0.22	0.25	mg/kg
Copper:	21.00	20.00	mg/kg
Manganese:	2.94	1.5	mg/kg
Nickel:	2.74	0.8	mg/kg
Selenium:	1.48	2.25	mg/kg
Zinc:	164.00	185.00	mg/kg

		Threshold Values	
Aluminium:	3.06	2.5	mg/kg
Cadmium:	0.12	0.25	mg/kg
Mercury:	0.12	0.4	mg/kg
Lead:	3.16	1.0	mg/kg

CHART 2

Name: Mr J.B.   Date: June 1997

	Your Results	**Recommended Values**	
Calcium:	541.00	400.00	mg/kg
Magnesium:	47.00	35.00	mg/kg
Potassium:	87.00	75.00	mg/kg
Iron:	47.00	30.00	mg/kg
Chromium:	1.92	0.8	mg/kg
Cobalt:	0.26	0.25	mg/kg
Copper:	23.00	20.00	mg/kg
Manganese:	3.01	1.5	mg/kg
Nickel:	2.46	0.8	mg/kg
Selenium:	2.33	2.25	mg/kg
Zinc:	174.00	185.00	mg/kg
		Threshold Values	
Aluminium:	1.44	2.5	mg/kg
Cadmium:	0.09	0.25	mg/kg
Mercury:	0.11	0.4	mg/kg
Lead:	1.72	1.0	mg/kg

Aluminium and lead went down, calcium, selenium and zinc levels rose and they had twins, a boy and a girl.

Zinc will often be deceptive, as a high zinc may appear to be present if the hair is growing very slowly due to zinc deficiency! Once some zinc in restored, although some zinc deficiency symptoms such as stretch marks, lank hair, white spots on the finger nails, acne, eczema, poor appetite, reduced sense of taste and smell and reduced libido may disappear, the hair will also grow faster so that upon retesting, the zinc in the hair will appear to have fallen! Also, with the increased stimulation and energy, the zinc will be being used elsewhere. But, with persistence, it will rise in the hair eventually!

Our own research at the University of Surrey shows very clearly a number of interesting points.

It would appear that most of the *hormonal treatments*, if continued for more than a few months, tend to raise the level of copper and lower that of zinc, and in some cases also to lower selenium, manganese and magnesium.

Bert Vallee of Harwood University Medical School has pointed out that during the *last trimester of pregnancy*, the zinc falls in the blood and the copper rises. When the copper reaches a certain ratio to the level of zinc, the phenomenon of birth occurs. In the last trimester, the placenta tends to pack with zinc, so the ratio of copper rises in the blood. Copper is a brain stimulant. To restore the balance after birth, the rat or rabbit mother (and usually any other mammal except the human) will consume the placenta, and it was found that within 96 hours, the zinc/copper balance in the mother was back to normal. This he wrote up in *Mineral Metabolism*, Volume II B, edited by Comar & Bronner, 1965.

Work by *Oberleas and Caldwell* at Wayne State University in the 1970's demonstrated that mother rats rejected their litter when zinc deficient. They retired to the far corner of their cage, and refused to feed or care for their young, who subsequently died. The same phenomenon was observed with the manganese deficient females.

The human placenta when tested by *Derek Bryce-Smith* in the UK, was found to contain between 360-600 mg of zinc. There is a good case to be made for supplementing zinc in the first few weeks after birth, *not least because the zinc deficient son may later have fertility problems from undiagnosed and long term zinc deficiency.* Adequate zinc levels in breast milk will be very important for the son's future fertility.

There is research to show (and our experience has confirmed) that post-partum depression and maternal rejection of the baby responds well to zinc and manganese supplementation. This also improves lactation, reduces the chances of sore/cracked nipples in the mother, and hastens healing of birth abrasions. Both mother and baby sleep better so fatigue is minimised. Work by *Carl Pfeiffer* also confirmed that maternal bonding was enhanced by zinc and manganese repletion. The zinc deficient baby, if this deficiency is not corrected, will be fed zinc-deficient breast-milk and will cry continuously and the whole cycle will continue.

It is therefore unfortunate that the fertility drugs, after the first few months, tend to drive up levels of copper. This will inevitably send the zinc levels down, as these two minerals compete for the binding sites. For this reason, babies conceived after fertility treatments are often miscarried or born prematurely. Bonding and lactation are also put at risk, so is future fertility. This is the way to create a never-ending problem.

To some extent, this can be made less likely by the administration of zinc throughout the treatment, also selenium, magnesium and manganese as indicated. However, we find that almost always when the woman is restored to health and normal mineral status, ovulation will be restarted naturally, and it will be unnecessary to use artificial hormones. We also often advise reflexology to be used together with nutrients, to restore ovulation without resorting to hormones. The reflexologist can work to strimulate the pineal and pituitary gland to enhance the production of the woman's own natural hormones.

We find restoring levels of zinc and other nutrients guards against pre-eclamptic toxaemia, malformation of the baby and hyperactivity, where this has been the history with a previous pregnancy/baby.

The same nutrients that are vital in pregnancy and lactation are also vital for male fertility.

Sometimes, copper or lead may be high for environmental reasons, often this is due to drinking water collecting metal off the pipes. Copper pipes have sometimes been joined with lead-containing valves. Sometimes there is a lead connecting pipe from the mains to the boundary stop-cock. Where the copper joins to the lead, there is likely to be corrosion, and lead and copper will be leaching into the water. We therefore offer to test the water also when levels are seen to be high in the hair. We can then advise on a jug filter for kitchen use if the contamination is not too heavy, or a whole house filter, or replacing the lead or the copper water pipes. ABS plastic is probably the piping of choice where water is acidic. Copper is very easily leached from the pipes. The legal limit for copper in the water is 3ppm. We find women tend to accumulate copper in their bodies at a lower level than this, however, sometimes where the water has only 0.2ppm. This may be to do with estrogen activity. Men also accumulate copper from water, although often they have less than their wives. Nonetheless, this will drive down their zinc and other trace minerals, and will affect sperm development.

Sometimes horrendous levels of lead are seen after the use of the hair dye "*Grecian 2000*". By checking the pubic hair we can tell that it has been absorbed through the scalp and is around the whole of the man's body. There is no way it can be kept away from the sperm beds once it is in the blood. We advise men to stop using this, and shampoo the hair frequently in the following 8 weeks. Then cut a fresh sample of hair that has grown out since discontinuation of use. During the 8 weeks, we suggest a toxic metal cleansing programme of Vitamin C, garlic, milk thistle, Vitamins B1 and B12, to remove lead that has been absorbed through the scalp. Henna in women's hair dyes can produce high copper levels, and this can be tackled in the same way.

Often quite high levels can still be seen, which may take some time to reduce. It is important that attempts at conception are delayed until the levels are back to normal to protect the future baby.

Very low levels of chromium, manganese, zinc, selenium and cobalt can be seen in diabetics, so we are hopeful that keeping levels of these minerals (all of which are needed for pancreatic function) within the recommended range will help to prevent gestational diabetes. So far we have not had a case of this developing, so it is possible this strategy is proving effective.

The benefits to the baby are very marked. The well nourished baby, who is not suffering from heavy metal toxicity or mineral deficiency, cries much less, and is more alert and responsive while awake, and sleeps more soundly. Their appetite is good, and they have strong resistance to infection.

• • • • • • • • • • • • • • • • • • •

Factors that research has found can exacerbate hyperactivity/autism/learning difficulties

From my experience, most hyperactivity is caused by heavy metals, or by nutrient deficiencies, often exacerbated by common environmental problems that enhance these two factors; either before birth or during the early years.

At Birth

1. Drugs given in childbirth. (Homeopathy can mitigate if given soon after the birth)
2. Lack of oxygen at birth. (May be due to lack of manganese. Manganese carries oxygen in the blood to the mitochondria of the brain cell.)
3. Cranial distortion at birth. (Cranial Osteopathy can mitigate after the birth)
4. Separation from mother/crying unattended in hospital nursery.
5. Possible contamination from powder on midwife's latex rubber gloves.
6. Contamination from organophosphate pesticide, possibly from flowers sent from florists.

Babyhood

7. Early weaning. (Cow's milk/sugar allergy may develop)
8. Vaccinations/fever/convulsions. (Homeopathy can mitigate after event)
9. Early mixed feeding. (Food Allergies can develop due to immature digestive tract.)
10. Urinary tract infection. (Possible GUI from birth canal - use homeopathy)
11. Middle-ear infection/glue ear. (Possible GUI from birth canal - use homeopathy)
12. Gastro-enteritis. (Possible GUI from birth canal - use homeopathy)
13. Lung infections. (Possible GUI from birth canal - use homeopathy)
14. Early separation from mother. (This is traumatic for baby)

Childhood

15. Fluorescent lighting as in schools. (Can be replaced with full spectrum daylight lighting)
16. Trace mineral deficiencies. (Hair analysis and supplements)
17. Heavy metal contamination. (Hair analysis and supplements)
18. Organophosphate pesticides (Eat Organic)
19. Chlorine, nitrates etc in water. (Filter, or drink bottled. If contamination is heavy, bath water may be affected. Consider whole-house filter.)
20. Fluoride in water. (Drink bottled)
21. Food additives and salicylates, ie aspirin. (avoid)
22. Excess sugar in diet. (avoid)
23. Passive smoking. (avoid)
24. Gut parasites. (If in doubt, ask nutritionist to arrange stool test)
25. Aluminium vegetable pans at school.

Dentistry (Choose your dentist carefully)

26. Mercury amalgam dental repairs. (Do not allow child to have these)
27. Conventional orthodontistry, palate cramping. (Insist on palate widening by cranial osteopathy)

• • • • • • • • • • • • • • • • • •

So what do we do about all this Mineral Mayhem?

Toxic Metals

a. We try to eliminate the sources of the toxic metals.

b. The cessation of smoking and alcohol will do a lot for us.

c. We can offer testing facilities for anything you feel it may be a good idea to test - tap water, any medication - including herbs that you are taking, shampoos, tea bags, cosmetics, dust from home and workplace, etc.

d. We suggest a cleansing programme, which will include counter-balancing minerals such as calcium, zinc and selenium, and a tablet (containing Vitamin C, B1, B12 and garlic, apple pectin and a small amount of milk thistle) for cleansing.

e.   We also suggest eating peas, beans, lentils, garlic and onions for their cleansing properties and putting a cupful of cider vinegar in a warm bath and soaking in it, once a week for a couple of weeks.

Essential Nutrients

a.   We supplement the mineral which is low, with a view to building the levels up to the optimum for the future pregnancy.

b.   We also give the synergistic mineral, if this is necessary, ie if the level is such that the extra metabolic activity would be likely to drop it below the optimum.

c.   We may also give competing minerals if the level makes it likely they would be reduced below the optimum by competition for the binding sites (ie when we give calcium we have to give magnesium. When we give zinc, we have to give selenium or these minerals would go down too far.)

A number of factors can influence the optimum uptake of trace minerals, and a number can make the levels go down rather than up in the hair.

When I am asked "Why have my levels gone in the wrong direction?" this is my reply:
The human body is quite volatile, and the levels of trace minerals are in a constant state of flux. Each meal, and with some minerals each breath, brings a fresh influx, and minerals are lost in outward breath, perspiration, urination and bowel movements.

Minerals are carried round the body by the blood and lymph, and all the body fluids vary round the day, which is why hair is the most stable sample for information on mineral status.

The hair gathers available minerals from the blood, which is transporting minerals around the body; excesses and paucities are therefore quite well reflected in the hair. A sample about an inch long reflects the mineral history of the previous 6-8 weeks, which makes it quite a stable reading, as it is not fluctuating and altering every few hours, as with blood, sweat, urine, saliva etc.

However, we all need to be aware of some aspects of hair analysis.

a.   If the supplements significantly enhance the health of the person taking them, this may increase the rate of growth of the hair. Faster growing hair may contain somewhat lower levels of some of the minerals we are looking at. This is, in fact, likely to be a more valid reading of the body status, than the more optimistic levels shown in the reduced growth of the first sample! Further supplementation can achieve good levels even in the normally growing hair. These are then the optimum levels for a healthy pregnancy.

b.   If there has been a high level of a toxic metal - lead, cadmium, mercury or aluminium - or an over-high level of the essential mineral copper - you will have been given 2-6 "Vitamin C with Garlic" to take it down. This can tend to take other minerals down also. This will be partly due to enhanced bowel actions, which may hasten the transit time of the food. It will also owe something to the ability of the body to coat (chelate) the toxic substances with a non-toxic substance such as zinc or selenium to carry them safely through the liver and kidneys and out of the body. This will mean that, even though we have given some zinc and selenium, these may also have gone down along with the toxins.

c.   It is the policy of the body to store any toxic metal it is exposed to in large quantities, until such time as circumstances are more favourable to cope with the overload. When B complex vitamins and minerals such as zinc, selenium, manganese, calcium etc, enter the body, sometimes these cells start to evacuate larger stores of lead, cadmium, mercury etc into the blood. This will take some months, rather than weeks, to clear, so the second hair chart may show some dumping of toxins. The more that is released the better, as the quicker we can get it to leave the body, the better. However, be very careful not to become pregnant until this has been fully achieved as all of the toxic metals, if present in large amounts, can cause health problems with the baby.

Do not be tempted to leave the metals "in storage" however, as in response to pregnancy hormones they would be released into the body, and could not be kept away from the developing embryo.

Sadly, we often see high levels of toxic metal in people who have come to us after the birth of a malformed baby. If only this work was done with one and all routinely, so much suffering could be avoided.

d.   The body has ways of trying to balance the levels of the minerals so that no single one will predominate in the body. Zinc, selenium and manganese all share binding sites in the intestine. You therefore need to take a little of one when you take any other of these (ie if you are taking zinc, you need to balance it with a little selenium, even if the selenium does not show a low level in this reading, or it will go down). Magnesium will enhance the utilisation of calcium, so giving either, without enough of the other, can result in the levels of the neglected element going down. It is not always an easy matter to get the balance exactly right, and we can sometimes struggle for several programmes. A lot may depend on the levels of lead, copper etc, in the drinking water and even the house dust, and nutrients in the diet. Levels are often slow to rise in people who do not give up alcohol.

Increasing the rate of growth of the hair, mobilising previously stored toxic metal, activating previously sluggish enzyme systems, activating toxic metals leaving the body etc, can all, at least for a time, confuse the picture in the hair.

As you may have gathered, it is not always easy to achieve perfection in a short space of time! This is why it is unwise to take a hair analysis to an inexperienced person for interpretation. You can understand why they may be nonplussed or dismissive!

Hair reading has, however, down the years, proved a most worthwhile exercise in creating the elusive baby. I would not work without it. I let the results speak for themselves!

The babies who are ultimately born free from a toxic load of dangerous substances, and able to use any vitamin or mineral they require for their mental and physical integrity, are, unsurprisingly, perfectly formed and mentally and emotionally exceedingly bright.

1 have devoted my life to making it possible for you to achieve this, because I feel it is worth it. Be patient. We will get there.

CHAPTER 8

ENVIRONMENTAL TOXINS & ELECTROMAGNETICS

My thanks to Daphne May, industrial toxicologist, for this list.

Among the main bug-bears working against the sperm development are lead, cadmium, mercury, aluminium, tobacco, alcohol, street drugs, pesticide, fluoride and xeno-estrogens. There are also a whole host of industrial and medical products. These include:

1. **Lead used in making storage batteries and paints:**
   Fewer sperm, sperm that moved more slowly than normal (decreased sperm motility), and more funny shaped sperm (increased malformation of sperm).

2. **DBCP (dibromochloropropane) a soil fumigant now banned:**
   Mutagen, lowered sperm count, testicular dysfunction.

3. **Ionising and non-ionising radiation, the former found in nuclear plant and medical facilities, the latter in high voltage switchyards and in communications facilities:**
   Possible damage to sperm cells and lowered fertility.

4. **Anaesthetic Gases:**
   Unexposed female partners are thought to have higher than normal number of miscarriages.

5. **Vinyl Chloride used in plastic manufacturing:**
   Unexposed female partners are thought to have more miscarriages and stillbirths.

6. **Kepone used as pesticide:**
   Possible loss of sex drive, lowered sperm count and slower movement of sperm.

7. **Heat stress occurring in foundries, smelters, bakeries and farm work:**
   Lower sperm count and sterility.

8. **Carbon Disulphide used in the manufacture of viscose rayon and as a fumigant:**
    Possible loss of sex drive, impotence and abnormal sperm.

9. **Estrogens used in the manufacturing of oral contraceptive:**
    Possible loss of sex drive and enlarged and sore breasts.

10. **Methylene chloride used as a solvent in paint strippers:**
    Possible very low sperm count and shrunken testicles.

11. **EDB (Ethylene Di-Bromide) used as an ingredient in leaded petrol and as a fumigant on tropical fruit for export:**
    Possible lower sperm count and decreased fertility in wives of workers.

A recent update on mercury condensed from an article by dentist Dr Victoria Lee:

Mercury is capable of producing infertility, birth defects, problems with the foetus and abortion. We are most likely to encounter it in our mouths, via our dental repairs.

The body has an ability to tolerate mercury, it sits in the liver and kidneys. Most people can continue to function with mercury stoppings, so long as their kidney function is not impaired. However, it is a cumulative toxin.

There is no safe level and quite tiny amounts can do a lot of damage. An amalgam filling contains about half a gram of mercury - enough to poison a ten acre lake, with the attendant food chain permanently. An average mouth has 9 amalgam fillings.

Until the 1960s, the dentists used a mercury that was less potent than that which is used today, which releases up to 50 times more mercury. Also, cavities used to be lined, so that the mercury would not transport through the dentine and out into the bone around the tooth. Now different linings are used containing a high copper alloy, so the patient not only gets mercury but also a higher copper, both of which are contra-indicated for fertility.

For most people, the only exposure to metallic mercury is from fillings. It has been shown that 90% of the body's burden (which impacts on sperm development) is from metallic mercury. The remaining 10% is from organic mercury, which comes from fish and other sources.

The mercury from dental work travels into the lungs, and inhaled mercury vapour goes up through the head. The amalgam fillings also create an electrical current with other metals in the mouth. The saliva forms an electrolyte, this leaches out mercury from the fillings which is continuously swallowed. In the gut, the mercury is capable of changing the gut flora and creating antibiotic resistant bacteria. The bacteria at the gum margin can change the metallic mercury into methyl mercury, and again this will be swallowed.

Dental fillings must be removed very carefully, using a rubber dam. Unless great care is taken, vapour from the drilling out gets inhaled, and saliva contaminated and swallowed. The patient should breath other air by protecting the mouth with an oxygen mask. Regulations on how best to protect the patient are laid down by the International Academy of Oral Medicine and Oral Toxicology.

Removal of the fillings goes some of the way, however, it does not remove mercury left in the body or even in the jaw. Large amounts will be in the bone. Hidden mercury can be found under crowns and in root canal fillings. This mercury can go down through the tooth and into the bone.

To detoxify from mercury, we need to look at several aspects. We need to support cellular function and replace the missing nutrients. Zinc, selenium and Vitamin C are recommended along with sulphur based proteins such as whey powder. These form a complex by which mercury can leave the body.

We suggest that you ask your dentist to check for mercury leakage. Any new fillings should be mercury-free - not glass ionomers but white composite. Make sure the dentist is familiar with all the correct procedures.

Fluoride Update
Condensed from an article by Walter Graham

Fluoride causes miscarriages, stillbirth and genetic damage. Numerous studies world-wide show that in fluoridated water areas, there are higher numbers of hip fractures. Studies from the USA have also shown higher numbers of women's cancers and of Down's Syndrome babies. Fluoride interferes with the immune system and kidney function.

A Chinese study has shown that fluoride can penetrate the foetal blood/brain barrier and settle in cerebral tissue before birth, thereby affecting children's intelligence. IQ may be reduced by 5 to 19 points.

Fluoride has the same detrimental effects as mercury and has an affinity for it. It can take mercury from fillings and delivers this and other toxic metals to accumulate in the brain.

Fluoride is present in dental products, unleaded petrol, pharmaceuticals, factory waste, and some drinking water. Fluoride is an enzyme poison in the same class as cyanide. In the USA it is used as a cockroach powder and a rat poison.

The Environmental Protection Agency in Washington DC has reviewed papers over 11 years, including animal and human epidemiology studies and have concluded there is a causal link between water fluoridation and cancer, genetic damage, neurological impairment and bond pathology. They were particularly concerned to note the link between fluoride exposure and lower IQ in children.

In England, the symptoms and risks set out by the BMA include slow poisoning or fluorosis along with brown discolouring of the enamel of developing teeth, based on prolonged intake of water with 2ppm fluoride.

According to the World Health Organisation, at 3ppm, there are visible bone changes. Levels over 8ppm may lead to bone disorders and degenerative changes in the heart, central nervous system, reproductive system, kidneys and adrenals.

Fluoride has never been before the MCA to be assessed as a drug. It only stands before the Cosmetic and Toiletry Association, which does not require a margin of safety.

Avoid fluoridated water and fluoride toothpaste. Do not give fluoride tablets to children. Read labels and avoid products containing fluoride.

Hair Dyes

Well, we know, I think, that none of you ever dye your hair? Or do we? Perish the thought that I would ask you to disclose this! Nevertheless, (and in any case to warn your partner, if need be) it is as well to realise that many of the permanent hair dyes are fairly problematic stuff.

Apart from skin burning and irritation, and other local allergic reactions, these products can cause breathing problems, damage to the immune system which can result in rheumatoid arthritis, and even more seriously, bladder cancer. In the UK each year, there are more than 12,000 new cases of this cancer, and more than 4,850 deaths, over 1,600 of whom are among hairdressers. (Daily Mail, 17 April 2002, Tim Utton).

Not surprising then that at least 2 reports have listed birth defects among the many horrors. (The Independent, 17th April 2002, Jeremy Laurence)

Two particularly dangerous chemicals are: para-phenylenecliamine and tetra-hydro-6-nitro quinoxaline - watch the side of the box. (The Independent, 17th April 2002, Jeremy Laurence)

Hair dyes will remain on the scalp. With anything that touches the skin, up to 60% will be absorbed into the bloodstream. This will travel through the body, and the toxins will reach the testicles, and, in the woman, to the ovary. Later, if your partner has dyed hair, the unborn baby will be at risk from these chemicals.

Latterly a recognised problem in the unborn has been the inability to empty the bladder. On occasion, this has necessitated an operation while the baby is still in the womb. Could this be localised swollen tissue, caused by a bladder carcinogen in the mother's blood? More than half of all women in the UK dye their hair. (Evening Standard, 16 April 2002, Victoria Fletcher)

The take-home message about hair dyes - particularly the dark permanent dyes - is that they are bad news, so avoid them. Anything that is poisoning you, will also be poisoning the sperm. Realise that grey hair makes you look distinguished and experienced. Who wants to look young and callow? The fact you have hair is good news in itself, some of the chaps I ask for a hair sample tell me they are as bald as billiard balls! Be happy!

For your partner, rescue her from the pressures of the hairdressers and the advertisements which could be enticing her to an early grave or a childless future. Tell her she is beautiful as she could be with her own unique living real colouring - *because she is worth it!* (The money it saves may surprise you - £175 million a year is spent on hair dyes in the UK!)

If your partner is really unhappy with her own colour, despite all you say, there are some non-permanent, washout dyes that are, so far as we know at present, non toxic ie Herbatint from your local health store:

Green People:	01444 401444
Dr Hauschka:	01386 792642
Ren:	020 7935 2323
The Organic Pharmacy:	020 7351 2232
Farmacia:	020 7404 8808
Neal's Yard Remedies:	020 7627 1949

• • • • • • • • • • • • • • • • • •

Electro-magnetic Pollution

Also, we now discover, (as if the preceding was not quite enough!), there are problems with electro magnetic pollution. There are people who can pinpoint the sources, and there are some solutions to be had, but the experts are few and far between at present, and there may be waiting lists. Foresight can advise on an expert who can give your house a geophysical survey and advise you. At time of going to press their charge is £120 plus fares. At present, we would advise:

Things to be avoided in the house:

> **Mobile Telephones:**
> NB: it is particularly important for prospective fathers *not* to keep one in a trouser pocket, as they can be dangerous to the testicles. This could also be a cause of testicular cancer. NB: Use can cause brain cancer. Also, loss of brain cells. (I would avoid them *anywhere*!)

Microwave Ovens:
Have regularly checked for leakage of microwaves. Eat food cooked in it as seldom as possible. (Better still, don't have one at all!) Food

cooked in it is devoid of enzymes and vitamins. This is essentially useless food. I have also been told that food cooked in a microwave should be left for 4 minutes before eating, as it will otherwise microwave your stomach. This has been linked to stomach cancer. Another scientist has told me that microwaves travel at 186,000 miles per second, they do not hang around in food. Leave food to stand for them to get all the way through. Pre-prepared microwave meals are a nutritional disaster.

Electric Blankets:
Do not have it turned on once you are in the bed.

Luminous Clocks:
I have been told that you should not keep luminous clocks turned towards the bed at night. Preferably have one that is not luminous. In his book *Cross Currents*, Robert O Beckner, MD, states

> *"An electric clock plugged into a wall socket produces an amazingly high magnetic field because of the small electric motor that runs it. A small bedside alarm of this type will produce a field of as much as 5 to 10 milligauss two feet away. If the bedside table is placed close to the bed, so that the sleeper's head is within this range, the dose rate is considerable for the average eight hours per night. Battery operated clocks have a negligible field, and I recommend their use as substitute."*

VDUs, Electric Typewriters, TV Screens, etc:
It is possible to obtain a small device for checking the emission of radiation. Some household and office apparatus have quite heavy emissions. It is worth investigating if you are in regular contact.

Be aware of the back of those VDU's around you in an office, as they may be emitting more electromagnetism than the one you are using. Be aware also that the rays may travel through a wall, so do not position one backing onto your bedroom (or anybody else's bedroom!)

Do not surround yourself in any room with TV, hi-fi and computer station. Be very much aware of any pylons, mobile phone masts, etc. If they are within 500 yards of your home, have electro-magnetic fields tested. Foresight can advise on finding help.

Electro-magnetic pollution from natural Radon and Ley Lines

Attention seems to have been drawn to this area even more recently than to intestinal parasites!

I am interested (wary even) but not yet well informed.

I have gathered, however, that reaction can be damaging to chromosome structure in the baby. It is likely to be damaging to sperm. It can also cause miscarriage, leukaemia and cancer.

It is interesting to note that areas of high reproductive disasters are also areas where there is ancient granite substrata. Areas that would be prone to high levels of natural radon from any clefts in the granite.

For help to know whether your home has a high level of natural radon, contact The National Radiological Protection Board.

North:	01132 679041
South:	01235 831600

Other homes particularly at risk may be those that have pylons within sight of the windows, be within 2-3 miles of a nuclear power station, or be within a quarter of a mile of a mobile telephone mast, or an airfield with mobile radar screens. There is also the question of ley lines.

The following services are offered by Dr Patrick MacManaway of Whole Earth Geomancy, Westbank Natural Health Centre, Strathmiglo, Fife, KY14 7QP, Scotland. Telephone: 01337 868 945 or fax: 01337 860 233, who will willingly travel to anyone who is worried about electro-magnetic pollution affecting their health.

 Also Roy Riggs (01273 732523) and Roger Coghill (01495 752122) - see Useful Addresses. All do house visits at the time of going to press at about £120 per day plus fares.

Consulting Services

*   Rectification of geopathic zones
*   Assessment of background ionising radiation count
*   Assessment of background and local power frequency electromagnetic fields

If all this seems a bit fazing, see pages 189 to 191 for further clarification!

CHAPTER 9

WHAT SHOULD THE NATION DO?

RE: The Government. The UK needs:
The following is what Foresight would like to see happen. If you succeed in procreating, see if you can help with this. We need some fit, strong, determined men involved!

- **EC Quality Air**
  Lead and cadmium in even outdoor paint, and spraying with pesticides banned. Factory out-gassing emitting into water supplies, and chimney effluent rigorously monitored and controlled.

- **EC Quality Water Testing and Monitoring**
  No lead water pipes. Many copper pipes also replaced where water was contaminated above 0.2ppm. (How about the Army taking on the work of replacing these in peace time?).

- **Nitrates, Estrogens, Organophosphates** eliminated from use/ removed at reservoir level. *No fluoride.* Factory and farming effluent much more controlled (ie warble-fly treatments and sheep dip disposal organised centrally).

- **Food-unfriendly farm chemicals** banned, especially organophosphate pesticides.

- **Mercury Amalgams** substituted by white composite fillings and phased out.

- **Fluoride** banned everywhere, including toothpastes and tablets.

- **Food Additives.** A much reduced list, with those that promote illness banned. (see page 93 for list of safe additives agreed by all the experts involved.) Aspartame and MSG banned.

- **No Genetically Modified Foods** We have got on without them very well in the past. We do not know what horrors they may bring in the future. Over 90% of us have said we don't want them. The Government should ban them.

- **Natural Family Planning** taught in all the schools. Classes for adults available nationwide. To be used with barriers in the fertile phase if necessary. The contraceptive pill and the copper coil outlawed.

- **Nutrition and Mineral Metabolism** taught in all the schools. Advanced courses to A level standard. More courses in Universities and Medical Schools. A Chair in Mineral Metabolism at a University.

- **Organic Farming** encouraged by adequate subsidies. Agro-chemicals taxed a little more each year. Agricultural colleges asked to convert to organic methods. Only organic promotes health and is sustainable.

- **Organic Growing** of fruit and vegetables taught in all the schools. Produce to be used "in house". Surplus could be sold locally to swell funds.

- **Pre-Pregnancy Health Checks** including hair analysis, lifestyle advice, NFP instruction, GUI checking and treatment, and nutrient programmes to be available on the NHS.

- **Geophysical surveys** to detect electromagnetic pollution to be funded by Government. Land to be surveyed before permission for new building to be granted.

- **Allergy, Hypoglycaemia and Intestinal Parasites** studied in all Medical Schools.

- **Genito-Urinary Medicine Clinics** much more widely advertised, and where necessary, better equipped, ie microscopes that will reveal mycoplasmas and ureaplasmas. Perhaps more clinics. Preconceptual testing advised by NHS.

- **Cigarettes and Alcohol** to carry warnings regarding fertility, both male and female, and possible damage to the unborn baby from use immediately before and during pregnancy.

- **Advertising of Cigarettes and Alcohol** to be eliminated.

- **More Realistic Penalties for Drug Pushing** Drug crops to be routinely destroyed. Drug-making premises to be raided by police. More education on long-term mental, reproductive and emotional consequences. Effects on the unborn widely publicised.

- **More Conferring by Government Agencies with the Voluntary Bodies** to use, for the benefit of all, their expertise in their own particular field.

- **More research into effects of vaccinations.** A moratorium on vaccinations until an antidote has been found to eliminate the possibility of autism. Use of homeopathy to be researched.

- **All NHS Practices** to have "in house", and use or refer patients to, a nutritionist, a naturopath, a homeopath, an osteopath, a reflexologist, an acupuncturist, and a Natural Family Planning teacher, as appropriate.

- **Fertility Drugs and other Fertility Treatments** to be rigorously assessed regarding efficiency, short-term side effects and long-term side-effects on the mother, also for miscarriage, premature birth, malformation, baby deaths and for long-term effects on child development, mental, physical and emotional.

These are some of our ideas to make a better world for this small person to be born into. Make your own list as well and set to! Good luck!

Summary

As you will see from all of the preceding pages, in real life the problem of nutrient deficiencies, pollution, infection and electro magnetic stress, are not all separate and "boxable" items, each with a pill-popping solution, but are all interweaving parts of a living whole, which is different for every single person involved.

Your heredity, your parents' diet and health before you were born - which in turn would have depended, to an extent, on *their* parents' health before *they* were born . . . all has bearing.

What you have eaten, what you have drunk, what you have breathed in, what bugs you have caught, where they are situated in the body, what vices you have espoused, what pylons you live under etc, etc . . . it all adds up to your particular and unique problem.

Only You can be You. You can take concerted action to get things as good as you can. On the way to fatherhood you can become much fitter, stronger and even brainier - and this will be all to the good, as being a Family Man is very demanding!

The sperm beds are not an isolated area of the body. They are an integral part of You. If these cells are challenged by pollution, poor quality food, bugs and drugs, so is the rest of You. Your brain cells, your bone cells, your muscle cells, - all of you is "under the weather". The environment is against us, but we have the weaponry - and fight back we must. It is our life - we all need our virility, our vitality, our staying power, our brain power.

> This is the only life we have, this is the only chance of descendants we have, and this is the only planet we have. We need to fight back!

This is at a personal level. But at a national level - even at a planetary level - all of you out there pulling together as a Great Army fighting for New Life and Vital Health is something extraordinary and vital and inspiring.

So, in a nutshell . . .

In case you are thinking "*so what exactly do we do?*"

1. You optimise your diet.

2. You stop caffeine, smoking, alcohol and street drugs. Now!

3. You learn natural family planning, so your wife does not need to take oral contraception.

4. You trot round to the GUM clinic for a check up. Follow through until pristine!

5. You consider whether you may have an allergy, reactive hypoglycaemia or may have gut bugs. If in doubt, you take action to find out. You need a nutritionist. Foresight can help you.

6. You contact FORESIGHT, and have a hair analysis and follow advice to get your essential minerals up to speed and get rid of the toxic metals. We look forward to helping you.

7. You take steps to avoid electro-magnetic pollution. It is worth contacting the right person, and having a geopathic survey undertaken for your house, and perhaps for your place of work.

There is, according to our recent count-up, a 2 out of 3 chance that this is all you will have to do, and along will come junior. (It probably seems enough anyway!) Let us know when he/she arrives!

If you are not lucky within about a year, I would read the last part of this book and select an alternative practitioner in Section II.

We have tried to do our bit, by pulling together and presenting to you all we know. Good luck with your bit. I hope we have contact along the way. I hope you succeed. Foresight is there to help you. *Onward!*

Chapter 9

Alternative Ideas
Helpful People in the
Alternative Field

These are the basic recommendations we have been making to increase sperm count, their motility (keenness) and perfect development. We have been active in this area since about 1984. The first count-up we did we had an 81 % success rate. With a subsequent programme, with both males and females involved, we had an 86% success rate over all. Among these couples, 42% of the men were known to have had a reproductive problem at the outset. At very least, this gave a 66% success rate with the "infertile" males. It may have been higher, as they were not identified in the final count-up.

With our latest count-up of men with a fertility problem specifically, it came again to 66.2% of those who did all the programme.

So, in practice at least, 2 out of 3 people who have done this programme have had a baby. (Many have had more than one baby!)

However, there are some with whom we have not met with success, so we have felt we should look for further help for any left in this predicament. Some very kind and interested alternative practitioners have agreed to contribute their expertise, and I have been delighted to be able to add their contributions. Browse around Chapter 9 with interest, as I have, and take up anything you feel may be particularly helpful to you.

I am no expert in these particular areas, but they are all people I know and trust. If all is not solved by FORESIGHT, then this would be yet another "stone to turn".

Keep working on the case!

Reflexology
By Joan Bullock

5,000 years of Reflexology seems to confirm its value as a therapeutic technique. There is documented evidence in many areas to prove its worth and effectiveness. Reflex points have been charted so that there are specific points on the feet that refer to each and every part of the body.

The reflexes to the male reproductive glands - testes, prostate and vas deferens can all be manipulated on the feet by the reflexologist's experienced hands. This will increase blood flow to those areas of the body thus transporting more oxygen and nutrients to the reproductive organs. The lymphatic tissue reflexes can also be worked to help the removal of toxins, and transport of nutrients, and help with immunity against infection. Hormone levels can be balanced via the reflexes to the pituitary gland and testes, since it has a beneficial effect on all bodily fluids.

There is anecdotal evidence from clients and doctors to suggest that Reflexology increases sperm count and motility, although most men would not even be aware that Reflexology could help in this area.

Most people can appreciate the deeply relaxing effects of Reflexology, to combat stress. Stress has the effect of causing many physiological imbalances to the nervous system, the hormones, immunity, blood pressure and digestion. Clients seem to achieve a greater sense of well being and calm from weekly treatments of Reflexology. More intense treatment can be performed more frequently. Reflexology is a perfect combination with preconceptual nutrition, as it can improve digestion, absorption and waste elimination of food.

Homeopathy and Infertility
By Alan Crook

One of the main differences between the homeopathic and orthodox approaches is that Homeopathy treats the individual person, whereas orthodox medicine diagnoses and treats diseases. Thus there are not specific homeopathic cures for infertility, male or female. Each patient is interviewed in considerable detail and a remedy is worked out for him or her. The basis on which remedies are worked out is that a substance which can cause symptoms in a healthy person can cure those same symptoms in someone who is not healthy. An important part of professional homeopathic training is the study of remedies and of the symptoms which they can cause and therefore cure. Infertility is one symptom which may point to a disturbance in the patient's health.

The other main difference between those two systems of medicine is that, whilst orthodox medicine prescribes drugs in gross doses which have to be carefully regulated in order to avoid damage to the patient because of their toxicity, the potentised medicines used in Homeopathy are prepared in a way which dilutes the original substances well beyond a toxic level but enhances their energy field. All living beings possess an electromagnetic energy field which has been found to control life processes. If the resonance of this energy field is disturbed, resulting in illness, the energy of the correctly selected homeopathic remedy can rebalance this disturbance, leading to a restoration of health and redundancy of the symptoms. Thus, although the origin of a homeopathic remedy may be an extremely toxic substance, such as arsenic, lead, aconite or a snake poison, there is no danger of any toxic side-effects. Much scientific criticism of Homeopathy has focused on the absence of molecules in these very dilute remedies. From the chemist's point of view they can have no effect. However, scientists have recently discovered that when a substance is dissolved in water, clusters of minute ice-crystals are formed by electromagnetic energy. The structure of the crystals, viewed by electron microscopy, is unique to each substance dissolved, and the density of the clusters increases the more the solution is diluted and shaken up. Although that research had nothing to do with homeopathy, this is precisely the procedure followed in homeopathic pharmacy, and this discovery goes a long way towards explaining the so-called "memory of water", which has been ridiculed by many scientists in the past.

There is a branch of Homeopathy, known as Isopathy, by which any allergenic or toxic substance can be potentized by a homeopathic pharmacist and given to a patient to antidote something which has made them unwell, or to desensitise them to an allergen. However, true Homeopathy treats the whole patient. Whilst it is often possible to work out a remedy for oneself, in acute ailments or first aid situations, using one of the many home prescribing guides, when faced with a more deeply-seated problem such as infertility, it is wise to consult a fully-trained practitioner. College courses last 3-4 years, and usually include a strong element of human science as well as the philosophy and practice of Homeopathy, knowledge of the remedies, and much clinical training. Once in practice, the homeopath will seek registration with a professional association - the Society of Homeopaths is the longest established. This involved professional insurance and an undertaking to abide by the Codes of Ethics and Practice. At the time of writing there is no restriction on who may describe themselves as a homeopath - the title is not protected by law - so it is wise to check on training and qualifications when seeking out a practitioner for the first time. The Society of Homeopaths (2 Artisan Road, Northampton, NN1 4HU) can help you to find a qualified practitioner in your area and Yellow Pages are also helpful.

Most of us come into life with some inherited baggage, in terms of predisposition to certain types of illness (eg if either or both parents, and maybe a grandparent or two, suffered from allergies, hay fever, eczema, migraines or hyperactivity, the chances of the patient suffering from one of these conditions is high). One of Homeopathy's special strengths is that it can address such inherited susceptibilities at a constitutional level. Experience has shown that parents who receive constitutional homeopathic treatment not only become healthier themselves, but produce healthier children. Whilst the remedies do not damage the foetus if taken during pregnancy, clearly it is even better to enhance the parents' level of health before conception. Homeopathic treatment before conception is considerably enhanced if complemented by supplementation such as the Foresight programme, and this is doubly important if either partner is regularly exposed to environmental toxins, has a diet which is low in essential nutrients, or has a recent history of smoking, heavy alcohol consumption or use of the contraceptive pill. Homeopathy is about creating superior health on all levels, and clearly it will be hindered in its task if there are factors operating in the patient's life which continue to drag the health down. Other factors which can adversely affect health include spending long periods of time in strong electromagnetic fields (eg from overhead power lines or geopathic stress). A thorough homeopathic consultation will investigate all such possible adverse influences on the patient's health, and will also include questions about the family medical history, so be prepared!

To sum up then, Homeopathy is a powerful resource in the quest for a better quality of health on all levels, physical, emotional, and mental. It works gently because it adjusts the patient's energy rather than mounting a physical attack on germs or tissues. This is not to exclude the possibility that a well-selected remedy could stimulate a detoxification. Old conditions that might have been suppressed in the past may briefly re-appear on their way out as the remedy carries out its spring-cleaning duties. Should you decide to consult a homeopath for help with infertility, the remedy (or series of remedies) you are prescribed will be a remedy for you as a unique person, and not an "infertility pill". Your body, enjoying a higher level of health, should then begin to produce sperm of a higher quality, although it may need to be backed up by a suitable supplementation and possibly some changes in lifestyle or diet. A homeopathic practitioner will normally work in partnership with you, so that you share responsibility for the changes which will come about in your health. The World Health Organisation defined "health" (at Alma Ata, 1978) as *" . . . a state of complete physical, mental and social well-being; it is not merely the absence of infirmity or disease, . . . it is a fundamental human right."* Do take the time to seek out a well-qualified practitioner, and do remember that, whilst Homeopathy works swiftly in acute or life-threatening situations, chronic problems do not disappear overnight; the body takes time to adjust to changes.

Mahatma Gandhi said of Homeopathy (which is one of the major medical systems in use in India): *"Homeopathy . . . cures a larger percentage of cases than any other method of treatment, and it is beyond doubt safer and more economical and the most complete medical science."*

Homeopathy and Western Medicine
Healing techniques work by enhancing the normal healing ability of a person and removing anything that upsets health in the first place. The balance and timing of these two factors is important in restoring health.

In the last 200 years, Homeopathic medicine has developed alongside Western medicine but has been less well known. It is now recognised as complementary to other treatments and has the ability to deeply enhance the healing of people.

The Homeopathy we know today was developed by Dr Samuel Hahnemann in Europe in the 19th Century. As an experiment, he gave himself doses of Peruvian bark, to find out its effect. It was then being used as a treatment for malaria and Quinine was later made from it. To his surprise it caused malaria type symptoms in himself - an otherwise healthy person. This gave him the principle that a remedy causes symptoms in a healthy person similar to those it will treat in an ill person.

Western medicine has focused on eliminating symptoms to alleviate suffering and prevent early death and has given us treatments that may be essential when irreversible body changes have occurred.

Homeopathic medicine aims to promote our natural vitality and uses symptoms as a guide to treatment.

Consider the course of a fever without drug treatment. In the past the person would be given appropriate care and food and the fever watched. It was allowed to develop to a crisis, which is the turning point in the illness. If all went well, recovery then started. Homeopathic remedies speed up this healing process. The peak is reached in minutes or hours in acute illness and the body moves towards healing. There is relief from the worst symptoms, a calmer feeling generally and the body heals naturally.

In the long-term illness the process is slower but the same. The healing ability is enhanced so that the person proceeds to the end of the illness in a positive way. In this way homeopathic remedies assist a person to help themselves and can work alongside other treatments.

Homeopathic Medicines

These are usually called remedies to distinguish them from orthodox medicines. They can be made from many substances in nature and due to the way they are prepared, by dilution and succession, they do not give any toxic side effects.

They are selected for each person individually on the homeopathic principle of similarity of symptoms in remedy and illness.

When to consider Homeopathy
By Dr Moira Houston

This is written as a guide to the type of work that I do and is not intended as a comprehensive overview of homeopathic treatment. I feel that the practitioner is integral to the help offered and it is from whom we are that particular interests and specialities result.

I explore mind and emotion, family history, diet, environment etc, with patients and use the information to select remedies to help the integration and healing process on its way. Anyone could benefit from homeopathic treatment but to give a few indicators we can think of it in three categories.

A: **Early in illnesses and recurrent problems where simple supportive treatment is insufficient, for example:**

Recurrent otitis media or URTI (urinary tract infection), recurrent cystitis
Any post-infection debility
Migraine
PMS, Dysmenorrhea, Menopause
IBS (irritable bowel syndrome)
Post operative recovery (best started before the operation in fact)

Well chosen remedies to suite the person's constitution can clear up many of these problems remarkably quickly.

B: **Transition times in life, which are really healthy but may benefit from extra help, for example:**

Pregnancy - before, during and after.
Infertility 1' or 2' [see (D)]
Infancy and childhood - all stages.
Adolescence with menstruation, acne, exams etc.   Menopause
Job changes and retirement
Marriage, divorce or relationship breakdown
Shock or trauma following injury or witnessing accidents
Bereavement and approaching death

Remedies and discussion assist the transition and healing.

C: **Chronic Illness, which requires more treatment and may need drug support as well, for example:**

Gastrointestinal disease, Ulcerative colitis, Crohns disease, food intolerance.

Rheumatoid arthritis and other autoimmune disease.

Cancer, MS, Diabetes, Hypertension

Management of emphysema or bronchitis

Multiple sclerosis and other neurological disease - as a supportive treatment.

Early in the disease these can respond to solely Homeopathy and later it can make the regular drug treatment more effective, reducing dosages and side effects.

In these situations, I work with the patient to improve their ability to heal themselves and so this needs the patient to be motivated and involved in the process. The help I offer can facilitate this and even wake up new interest but in the end the patient is doing the healing mostly on a mental and emotional level. Remedies make a link from this to the physical illness. (Other Homeopaths may use different approaches.)

D: **Illness with a mixed physical, environment, allergic and emotional factors, such as:**

Skin diseases - eg Eczema, Psoriasis, Warts etc

Asthma, Bronchitis, Any chronic infection

ME and other illness where treatment is problematical

Infertility 1' or 2'

May need diet change as well as remedies and need other treatments.

Energy Balancing for Home and Office
By Dr Patrick MacManaway

Westbank Natural Health Centre, Strathmiglo, Fife, KY14 7QP.
Telephone: 01337 868945

Geopathic Stress and Infertility

Geopathic stress is a stress factor affecting humans, plants, birds and animals. It is a location-specific stressor, and occurs as a consequence of one of several mechanisms.

Firstly, geopathic stress may be caused by weak perturbations in the earth's' magnetic field. These are typically due to veins or aquifers of subterranean water, flowing in rock fractures tens or sometimes hundreds of feet below ground level, although dry fissures and fractures, cavities, mine workings, and deposits of crystals or minerals may have similar effect. Very occasionally, large diameter or high volume drainage channels may create such disturbance, although natural features are more frequently at issue. Secondly, other natural energetic features that are less well understood scientifically can cause geopathic stress. These include features such as ley-lines and "earth grids" - dowseable energy lines which correspond to the "dragon lines" of ancient China, carrying "chi" over the surface of the body of the earth in the same way that acupuncture meridians carry chi over the surface of the body of a person. These can have various direct and indirect effects on plant and animal health.

Thirdly, geopathic stress can be caused by "place memory" - the residue of human psychic and emotional residue that accumulates over time in any place where humans are present. Place memory can be either beneficial, neutral, or detrimental to health depending on its nature. Old battlefield sites and places that hold the memory of murder or rape can have very negative impact on the human psyche and emotional body. Fourthly, places may hold the spirits of the dead, "earth-bound" due to unresolved emotional attachment to the circumstances of their earthly lives. Needing loving attention and healing for their release into the light, they can create considerable psychic and emotional disturbance in their earth bound state. Nature spirits disturbed or dislocated by building-site construction can also cause similar problems of a psychic and emotional nature.

Geopathic stress and the various subtle energies of place can be worked with to bring peace and balance and to create a healthy environment in the majority of cases. Techniques for working with geopathic and related stress factors vary considerably from practitioner to practitioner. Many practitioners use dowsing as a tool of assessment and practice, and the British Society of Dowsers holds a register of such practitioners who make their services available to the public.

Geopathic stress can be diagnosed by thorough Vega testing, kinesiology, dowsing, and other subtle and intuitive systems, or may be apparent as a diagnosis if health problems have occurred following a move to a new home or work location. Geopathic stress is one of several location-specific stress factors which include electromagnetic field pollution from high-tension power lines, mains wiring, lighting rings, radio and microwave sources, radon gas pollution, air pollution from other volatile or airborne organic and inorganic compounds including asbestos, air pollution from air-conditioning systems, inadequate lighting, especially the absence or relative scarcity of natural sunlight, and psychological stress factors resulting from poorly arranged and dysfunctional work environments.

Geopathic stress affects the human body by disturbing the pineal glands' ability to detect the natural daily flux of the earth's magnetic field, resulting in a disorientation of the biological clock and subsequent disruption of biological cycles including the sleep cycle and menstrual cycle. Consequent difficulty in conception and in carrying a healthy pregnancy to full term is seen not only in affected women but also in horses, cows, sheep, pigs and goats. Geopathic stress can also have a detrimental effect on the health of any part of the body repeatedly exposed to a stress line, and if the pelvic area is influenced by a line of geopathic stress crossing the sleeping position in bed, pathology or dysfunction of the reproductive organs may result.

The World Health Organisation states that 30% of all buildings may be "sick buildings" based on the criteria that 20% of the occupants may be experiencing health or comfort problems. In buildings where this is the case, or if ill health has arisen following a move to a new home or work place, the presence of geopathic stress should be assessed, and appropriate remedial action taken if it is found to be present. Likewise new construction projects should ideally be assessed to ensure an appropriate and stress-free location is chosen.

Electromagnetic Field Stress and Infertility

The earth's atmosphere has for the period of human evolution been filled with weak, low frequency electromagnetic waves, primarily between the frequencies of 0-30 cycles per second. These "micropulsations" are created by the interaction between the solar wind - a stream of particles emitting constantly from the sun - and the ionosphere - a protective layer of the earth's atmosphere.

Due to the constant presence of these waves and their daily and seasonal fluctuations, the human brain and adrenal bodies have a well developed sensitivity to this field, and rely on it as one channel of sensory input from our surrounding environment.

Exposure to man-made electromagnetic fields of these and also higher frequencies emulate but in an exaggerated or distorted way those naturally-occurring frequencies, and can be shown to create changes both in mood and in physiology, causing the brain to release neuropeptides in the same way as though stimulated by psycho-active chemicals. Disturbance in the function of the pineal gland, with a consequent imbalance in serotonin and melatonin, is the primary physiological pathway for the effects of electromagnetic field pollution on the body, and the dysfunction of the biological time-keeping activities of this gland, which include the regulation of the sleep cycle and the menstrual cycle, can have a detrimental effect on human fertility. A secondary disturbance occurs due to the inappropriate function of the adrenal glands and disturbance in the normal stress response that they mediate.

Sources of electromagnetic field disturbance include high-tension pylons, mains electricity in the walls of home and office, fields from electrical appliances, and fields from radio and microwave transmission. The levels at which such fields have detrimental health effects are controversial and much disputed. It should also be noted that prolonged and repeated exposure to these fields is of likely concern to health, while brief and intermittent exposure is less likely to be harmful.

Electromagnetic fields have two components - the electrical field, which is the potential for electrical current to flow, and the magnetic field, which is the field created by electrical current as it flows. The electrical field is generally present at all times when electricity is present in a building, whether or not any appliances are being used, while the magnetic field is present only when an appliance is in use.

Inexpensive meters for measuring electric and magnetic fields are readily available and easy to use, and the primary strategy when dealing with electromagnetic field pollution is one of "prudent avoidance", meaning removing oneself to a safe distance from the source of the field.

Most electromagnetic fields in a domestic or office environment drop off rapidly from their point of origin, and removing all appliances that run on mains electricity to a distance of three feet or more from the resting position of the body during sleep is a sensible first step in prudent avoidance. It should be noted that electrical wires in the walls of a bedroom may be within three feet of the bed head, in which case either moving the bed, screening the field or installing a "demand switch" on the relevant wiring circuit - which isolates and removes all fields from the circuit when it is not being actively used - may be necessary.

Further information on electromagnetic fields and their effects on health can be obtained from:

Electromagnetic Hazard and Therapy
by Simon Best & Alasdair Philips

PO Box 2039 Shoreham by Sea BN43 5JD

Website: http://www.perspective.co.uk

APPENDIX I

GLUTEN FREE RECIPES

Basic Cake
4 oz butter
3 oz brown sugar
2 eggs
Flour: 2 oz rice flour, 1 oz cornflour, 1 oz potato flour
$^1/_2$ level tsp bicarbonate of soda
1 level tsp cream of tartar
Or with 3 oz oil instead of the butter, as above

Flavour - any of the following:
Ginger, Vanilla, Cocoa, Orange or Lemon Juice

For fruit cake add:
Organic dried fruit and/or
Chopped prunes and cherries (non dyed) and/or
Dates, walnuts, almonds
Almond paste* and strawberry jam

Almond paste: Small packet organic ground almonds, tsp brown vinegar. Make a paste with orange or lemon juice. Put in centre of cake before baking.

Pastry (for sweet dishes)
3 oz rice flour
1 oz ground almonds
2 oz potato flour
3 oz Trex or butter

Pastry (for savoury dishes)
2 oz rice flour
2 oz potato flour
2 oz Trex or butter

Roll and cook in the usual way (as best you can as it is very breaky!)

Shortbread
Mix 2 oz rice flour, 1 oz cornflour, 1 oz ground almonds, 1 1/2 oz brown sugar.
Knead in 2 1/2 oz butter.
Press down in baking tray, prick with a fork all over. Bake in a moderate oven for about 10 minutes. Take out and cut into squares while it is still soft. Then put back in oven for about 20 minutes more.

Jellies, junkets, tapioca, rice and cornflour puddings are all gluten free anyway, as is ice cream, and almost all yoghurts (but beware of "modified starch").

For a crumble topping for any form of stewing fruit, mix:
3 oz rice flour
3 oz cornflour
2 oz ground almonds
3 oz brown sugar

When thoroughly mixed, rub in 4 oz butter (if not milk allergic) or dribble in a little safflower oil and mix well.

Press down onto the cut-up fruit and bake for about half an hour.

Gravy and Brown Sauce, Gluten Free
Mix a dessert spoonful of cornflour with enough cold water to make a smooth, liquid mixture. Add boiling water. Add this thickened mixture to juices in the roasting pan, or boil in a saucepan with a gluten free stock cube (check this on the box) or Bovril, Marmite, or Yeast extract. A pinch of Brewer's Yeast powder can be added to supplement B-complex vitamins. To make a brown sauce for stews etc, proceed as above, using a little more cornflour and add onions, sweetcorn, garlic, Heinz tomato ketchup, sliced carrot, mushrooms, aubergine and/or courgettes etc. For pork, add sliced apple or prunes. For lamb add some gluten free chutney, (check label).

Rice can be added to stews in the place of pearl barley.

Gluten-free White Sauce - for those who are not milk allergic
Boil 1/2 pint of milk with a knob of butter or margarine, or a dessert spoonful of oil. Keep a little of the milk back and mix cold with a tablespoonful of cornflour. Add boiling milk and return to pan and boil until it thickens.

Savoury recipes

Add to this basic white sauce parsley for fish, grated cheese for cauliflower, mushrooms, onions for chicken, or ginger and apricot for posh chicken - whatever you wish! Grapes for sole. Add salt to taste.

Sweet recipes

Add maple syrup, honey or sugar free jam if you want a cornflour pudding. Marmalade, ginger and brown sugar, lemon and brown sugar and pour it over sponge pudding, or anything you like!

With milk allergy, rice dream (unflavoured) may be substituted for milk, and the oil option taken, but this is very bland, so you need plenty of flavouring. There is also goat's milk, oat milk or coconut milk.

Sponge Pudding

3 oz rice flour
1 oz cornflour
1 oz potato flour
3 oz brown sugar
4 oz butter
3 eggs
1 tsp gluten free baking powder

Add sultanas, and/or other dried fruit, syrup or jam at bottom of bowl, or mix in jam, chocolate, ginger, cinnamon, and steam it for two hours.

Or, put it as a topping on chopped fruit, and bake it in the oven

Pancakes - for once, nicer than glutinous!

2 oz rice flour
2 oz cornflour
1 egg
$1/2$ pint milk or water

SEE BOOK LIST FOR BOOKS TO HELP!

APPENDIX II

SURVEY OF PEOPLE WHO CONTACTED US OVER A PERIOD OF TWO YEARS WITH MALE INFERTILITY

This has not been an easy survey to pull together at all, as people do a number of different aspects of the programme and some more thoroughly than others, and each couple comes to us with a different range of health problems. In some cases the wife has health problems of her own, which may inhibit conception. We have, however, been as meticulous as possible, and I will try and present the findings as clearly as possible.

Between 1996 and 1998 we were contacted by 370 couples who had been told that the male infertility problem was so severe that donor sperm or adoption were their only options. This year, in anticipation of this book, we set out to complete the data by contacting again those who had not let us know the outcome to the programme.

Unfortunately, among them were 97 couples who had moved away and had not left a forwarding address, so we were unable to discover what had happened. This is not necessarily a negative outcome, as an unknown number may have moved because they needed extra space for a baby, but frustratingly we will never know. This left us with a population of 274 couples for the Survey. Of them, 68 couples told us they had not done the programme at all. Some said this was for reasons of expense, some because the idea had been ridiculed by their family or their GP, and one because "they did not feel dedicated enough". Of these 68 non-participating couples, 11 couples had achieved a live baby, or babies, totalling in all 13 babies and one ongoing pregnancy. (For the purposes of this research we are counting an ongoing pregnancy as one singleton live birth.) There had been 4 miscarriages and 1 stillbirth. There had been 2 attempts at IVF, and one of these had been successful. Also, one woman had had ovarian cysts treated and this couple had achieved twin boys.

196

Therefore the success rate for non-participants had been 16.2%. The number of babies per head of group population had been 20.1%. The success rate of IVF had been 50% (2 couples, 1 baby).

It is interesting to note that the HFEA Study concluded that the average success rate for IVF was 22.6% but that this group who did nothing achieved almost this rate without any assistance at all! If any doctor or researcher is reading this book, this first group being non-participants could be regarded as a "control population".

The remainder of the population, 209 couples, had done some aspect of the programme. The uptake had been very variable. On their own estimations, we asked them to tell us whether they had done the programme "Partly", (a small part), "Mostly", (a large part but with specific omissions), or "All of It". They filled in a questionnaire, and this was checked against their files for added accuracy.

Results
Adding up all of the couples (209) who did any part of the programme, 107 of these couples have achieved at least one baby and/or ongoing pregnancy, (52.4%). All told, 119 babies and 15 pregnancies at the time of going to press (65.7% babies per head of the population).

So how did the population divide up? There were 47 "Partly People", 18 "Mostly People", and 139 who claimed they did "All of It".

"Partly" People
Ten couples from the 47 in the "Partly" group had achieved between them 10 babies and 2 ongoing pregnancies. Sadly, there had also been 7 miscarriages in the "Partly" group.

A success rate for couples of 21.3%. Children per head of population 25.5%.

From the "Partly" group, 4 couples went for IVF. One couple achieved twin girls. One other woman was pregnant at the end of the survey.

IVF success per couple - 50%. 3 babies from 4 treatments - children per head of population 75%!

"Mostly" People
Only 18 couples said they had done the programme "Mostly". Most usual crucial omissions were the GUI check and/or male abstention

from alcohol. There were 5 successful couples, who have 5 babies and 1 ongoing pregnancy between them.

A success rate of 27.8% for couples. Children per head of population, 38.9%. Nobody in this group went in for high-tech. There were no miscarriages in this group, but one couple, where the mother had diabetes, had a stillbirth. This birth is not included in the above figures.

"All of it" People

139 couples said they had done "All of It". Of these, 92 couples have achieved a live birth or had an ongoing pregnancy, (66.2%). Almost exactly 2 out of 3 couples. These couples had achieved between them 103 babies and 12 ongoing pregnancies. Children per head of population, 82.7%. There were also, sadly, 3 miscarriages.

12 couples in this "All of It" group went in for IVF or other high-tech treatments. 9 of these couples achieved success and 4 had failures (9 failures). One mother failed IVF, and then had a further attempt which achieved a daughter, followed by another which achieved an ongoing pregnancy, so this mother fell into both categories. Other participants fared as follows:

IVF:	One girl baby
IVF:	Twins, a boy and a girl
IVF:	Twins, a girl and a boy
IUI:	Twins, a boy and a girl
3 IUI followed by 3 IVF:	No baby
ICSI:	Twin girls (father has no vas deferens)
IVF:	No baby
IVF:	No baby
Clomid Only:	Twin girls
IVF:	Twin boys

SUCCESS PER TREATMENT: 50%

3 couples are still childless from this group.

Miscarriage and stillbirth rate between the four groups

No programme undertaken: 4 miscarriages   (5.9%)
47 "Partly" people: 7 miscarriages   (14.9%)
18 "Mostly" people: 1 stillbirth   (5.5%)
139 "All of It" people: 3 miscarriages   (2.2%).

Demonstrating how greatly improved the outcome if the programme is fully completed.

These outcomes are summarised for you in the following chart:

Category	Not At All	Partly - small part	Mostly - omissions	All Of It
Total Couples	68	47	18	139
Couples achieving live birth or ongoing pregnancy	11 (16.2%)	10 (21.3%)	5 (27.8%)	92 (66.2%)
Number of births and pregnancies	13 births 1 pregnancy (20.1%)	10 births 2 pregnancies (25.5%)	6 births 1 pregnancy (38.9%)	103 births 12 pregnancies (82.7%)
Miscarriages	4	7	0	3
Stillbirths	0	0	1	0
Babies born by high tech	IVF 1 baby cysts treated twin boys	1 pregnancy twin girls	no high tech used	6 pairs twins 2 singletons 1 pregnancy
High tech failure	3 (60%)	2 (50%)	- -	9 (50%)
Couples with no high tech	65	43	18	128
Babies no high tech	11 (16.2%)	9 (19.1%)	7 (38.9%)	90 (71.4%)

NB "Pregnancy" means this pregnancy was still ongoing when the study ended.

Average Weights

No part of programme: Only one couple gave weights. In their case the husband did not do any part of the programme *but the wife did it all!* They had a boy, 8lb 13oz and a girl 9lb 1oz. Average weight was 8lb 15oz.

Small part of programme: 4 weights were given. Single babies: Average weight 7lb 2oz. Twin babies: Weight was given for one pair as 6lb and 7lb. Average twin weight was 6lb 8oz.

Most of programme: Only 4 weights were given. Single babies: Average weight 8lb 1oz. No twins in this group.

All of It: All weights were given. Single babies: Average weight was 7lb 9oz. Twin babies: Average weights 5lb 1oz.

Of the couples who have succeeded so far, while taking at least a part or all of the programme: 10 are on their first pregnancy, 70 have had just one child, 10 couples have had twins, and 11 have had more than one singleton child or are on their second pregnancy - two mothers are on their third pregnancy!

So be happy, it could work for you too! Our thoughts are with you.

APPENDIX III

RECOMMENDED SCIENTIFIC RESEARCH
Papers that lie behind the FORESIGHT philosophy

- **Alder, MW**, ABC of Sexually Transmitted Diseases, London, BMA 1984, 48
- **Ali Brac De La Perriere, Robert & Seuret**, Franck (2000), Brave New Seeds, The Threat of GM Crops to Farmers, Zed Books
- **Anon**, (1993), Pregnancy and Exposure to Alcohol and Other Drug Use, US:DHHS
- **Anon**, Food Irradiation Facts, National Coalition to Stop Food Irradiation, San Francisco, CA, undated
- **Anon**, Oregon Enacts America's First Law to Diagnose Underlying Organic Causes of Mental Illness, Int J Biosocial Res, 1984, 6(1), 13
- **Ashton, Professor CH**, (2001), Benzodiazepines, UK Edition Vol 8
- **Baird Cousins**, 'Effects of Undernutrition on Central Nervous System Function', Nutr Reviews, 1965, 23, 65-68.
- **Balfour, EB**, The Living Soil and the Haughey Experiment, New York, Universe Books, 1976,29
- **Ballentine, Rudolph**, Diet and Nutrition, Honesdale, PA The Himalayan International Institute, 1978, 72.
- **Barlow, SM, Sullivan, FM**, Reproductive Hazards of Industrial Chemicals, London, Academic Press Inc, 1982, 40
- **Bell, Margaret,** (2002) Living with a lethal legacy - The appalling damage prescribed drugs are causing our children, The Lantern
- **Bellinger, David et al**, 'Longitudinal analyses of prenatal and postnatal lead exposure and infant development in the first year' New Eng J Med, 1987, 17, 1037-1043
- **Bellinger, David et al,** 'Low-level lead exposure and infant development in the first year' Neurobehavioral Toxicol and teratol, 1986, 8, 151-161
- **Best, Simon,** (2000), Microwave Ovens - A Recipe for Disaster, What Doctors Don't Tell You, Vol 10, No 12
- **Birkin, Michael & Price, Brian,** (1989), C for Chemicals - Chemical Hazards and How to Avoid Them, Green Print
- **Blair, J H. et al,** 'MAO inhibitors and sperm production' JAMA, 1962, 181, 192-193
- **Blather, Russell J,** 'The role of viruses in congenital defects' Am J Dis Child, 1974, 128, 781-786
- **Bonnell, JA,** 'Physical Hazards', In: Dizon, WM. Price, Susan MG. eds. Aspects of Occupational Health, Faber and Faber, 1984, 167-194.

- **Brett, Mary,** (2002), Maranatha Workshop - The Adverse Affects of Cannabis
- **Brett, Mary,** (2003), Cannabis and its Affects, FORESIGHT Seminar
- **Bryce-Smith, D,** Environmental Influences on Prenatal Development, Thessaloniki Conference September 1981
- **Bryce-Smith, D, et al,** 'Lead and cadmium levels in stillbirths'. Lancet 1977, 11159
- **Bryce-Smith, D,** 'Environmental trace elements and their role in disorders of personality, intellect, behaviour and learning ability in children'. Proceedings of the second New Zealand Seminar on Trace elements and Health. University of Auckland, 22-26 January 1979.
- **Bryce-Smith, Derek, Hodgkinson, Liz,** 'The Zinc Solution', London, Century Arrow 1986, 28-29
- **Bryce-Smith, Derek, Hodgkinson, Liz,** 'The Zinc Solution', London, Century Arrow, 1986, 33-38
- **Buist, Robert,** 'Drug-Nutrient Interactions', International Journal of Clinical Nutrition
- **Bunyard, Peter, Morgan-Grenville, Fern,** eds. The Green Alternative, London, Methuen, 1987,83
- **Bushnell, Philip J, Bowman, Robert E,** 'Reversal learning deficits in young monkeys exposed to lead', Pharmacology Biochemistry and Behaviour, 1977, 10, 733-747
- **Caldwell, Donald F, Oberleas, Donald,** 'Effects of Protein and Zinc Nutrition on Behaviour in the Rat'. Perinatal Factors Affecting Human Development, 1969, 185, 2-8
- **Cannon, Geoffrey,** 'Why Hampstead Babies are 2 lbs Heavier', The Sunday Times, 28th March, 1983.
- **Cannon, Geoffrey, Walker, Caroline,** The Food Scandal. London, Century Aitow 1986: 121-154
- **Cannon, Geoffrey,** The Politics of Food, London, Century, 1987
- **Carlsen, H, Guverman, A. et al,** 'Evidence for decreasing quality of semen during past 50 years.' BMJ 305: 609-13.
- **Catterall, RD,** 'Biological effects of sexual freedom'. Lancet, 1981, 315-319
- **Chaitnow, Leon,** 'Candida Albicans. Could Yeast Be Your Problem?' Thorsons, 198, 48.
- **Chattopadhyay, Amares et al,** 'Scalp hair as a monitor of community exposure to lead'. Arch Anviron Health, 1977.
- **Churchill, John A, et al,** 'Birth Weight and Intelligence', Obstet Gynecol, 1966, 28, 425-429.
- **Coghill, Roger,** (2003), Do High Voltage Powerlines Affect Vicinal Earthworm Populations? Coghill Research Laboratories, Gwent
- **Colquhoun, Irene, Barnes, Belinda,** 'The Hyperactive Child. What The Family Can Do', Wellingborough, Thorsons, 1984.

- **Crawford, IL, Connor, JD,** 'Zinc and Hippocampal Function'. J Orthomolecular Psych, 1975, 4(1), 39-52
- **Crook, William G,** The Yeast Connection, Professional Books, 1983
- **Cross, Douglas,** (2003), Fluoridation - Unlawful Poisoning, Environmental Issues Forum Newsletter
- **David, Oliver J et al,** 'Lead and hyperactivity. Behavioural response to chelation: a pilot study', Am J Psychiatry, 1976, 133(10)1155-1158
- **Davies, Stephen and Stewart, Alan,** Nutritional Medicine, London, Pan, 1987, 360
- **Davis, Adelle,** 'Let's Eat Right To Keep Fit', New York, New American Library, 1954, 58.
- **Davis, Adelle,** 'Let's Have Healthy Children', Unwin Paperbacks, 1974, 26
- **Davis, J, et al,** 'Effects of phenelzine on semen in infertility: a preliminary report' Fert Ster, 1966, 17, 221-225
- **Department of Health,** 'Folic Acid and the prevention of neural tube defects: report from an expert advisory group', Heywood: DoH Health Publication Unit, 1992, 21.
- **Eagle, Robert,** Eating and Allergy, Wellingborough, Thorsons, 1986
- **Editorial:** 'The Drugged Sperm', British Medical Journal, 1964, l, 1063-1064
- **Erichman, James,** Gluttons for Punishment, London, Penguin 1986, 242
- **Fano, Alix,** (1997), Lethal Laws, Animal Testing, Human Health & Environmental Policy, Zed Books
- **Fine, PEM, et al,** 'Infectious diseases during pregnancy: a follow-up study of the long-term effects of exposure to viral infections in utero. Studies on medical and population subject' HMSO, 1985
- **Fletcher, David J,** 'Hair Analysis: Proven and problematic applications'. Postgrad Medicine, 1982, 72(5), 79-88.
- **Fletcher, David,** 'Scourge of the Sick Building Syndrome', Daily Telegraph, 24th March 1988
- **From the UK Councillor,** (1996), Issues of Democracy, Government accused of "dirty tricks"
- **Gal, Isobel, et al,** 'Vitamin A in relation to Human Congenital Malformations', 149.
- **Garraway, James L,** 'Trace Elements in Agriculture' Trace Elements in Health, Rose, J, ed. London Butterworth
- **Gittleman, Rachel, Eskenazi, Brenda,** 'Lead and Hyperactivity revisited', Arch gen Psychiatry, 1983, 40, 827-833
- **Glasser, George,** (2000), Fluoridation - A Mandate to Dump Toxic Waste in the Name of Public Health, The Safe Water Coalition, San Jose, California
- **Gordon, Garry F,** 'Hair Analysis: Its Current Use and Limitations. Part II'. Let's Live, October 1980, 89-94.
- **Grant, ECG,** Food Allergies and Migraine, Lancet, 1979, 1, 966-968

- **Griffiths, Joel, Bryson, Chris,** (1997), Fluoride, Teeth and the Atomic Bomb, NPWA
- **Hambridge, K, Michael et al,** 'Low Levels of Zinc in Hair, Anorexia, Poor Growth and Hypogeusia in Children'. Paediatric Research 1972,6,868-874
- **Hansen, J et al,** 'Children with minimal brain dysfunction', Danish Medical Bulletin, 1980, 27(6), 259-262
- **Hare, Francis,** The Food Factor in Disease, 1905
- **Hawkins, David, Pauling, Linus,** 'Orthomolecular Psychiatry, Treatment of Schizophrenia', San Francisco, CA, W.H. Freeman and Company, 1973.
- **Health Education Council,** A discussion paper on proposals for nutritional guidelines for health education in Britain. Prepared for the National Advisory committee on Nutrition Education by an ad hoc working party under the Chairmanship of Professor V.P.T. James, NACNE, September 1983.
- **Hefferon, David,** (2003), Mercury in Preconception and Pregnancy, FORESIGHT Seminar
- **Hemsworth, BN,** 'Deformation of the mouse fetus after ingestion of nicotine by the male', IRCS Medical Science; Anatomy and Human Biology; Biochemistry; Developmental Biology and Medicine; Drug metabolism and Toxicology; Pathology; Pharmacology; Physiology; Reproduction; Obstetrics and Gynaecology. 1981. 9, 727-9
- **Hill, Stuart B,** 'Soil Conditions and Food Quality' Undated paper by author, MacDonald College of McGill University.
- **Holiverda-Kuipers, J,** 'The cognitive development of low birthweight children', J Child Psychology and Psychiat, 1987, 28, 321-328.
- **Howell, Edward,** Food Enzymes for Health and Longevity, Woodstock Valley, Connecticut, Omangod Press, 1980, 5
- **Hurley, Lucille A,** 'Zinc Deficiency in the Developing Rat'. Am J Clin Nut, 1969, 22, 1332-1339
- **Hurley, Lucille S et al,** 'Teratogenic effects of Magnesium Deficiency' J Nut, 1976, 106, 1254-1260
- **Hurley, Lucille,** 'Developmental Nutrition, Englewood Cliffs, NJ, Prentice-Hall, 1980.
- **Hurley, Lucille, S,** 'Developmental nutrition', Englewood Cliffs, NJ, Prentice-Hall, 1980, 150.
- **Jacob, Martha et al,** 'A forgotten factor in pelvic inflammatory disease: infection in the male partner'. British Medical Journal, 1987, 294, 869
- **Jameson, Sven,** 'Zinc Status and Human Reproduction'.'. In; Zinc in Human Medicine. Proceedings of a Symposium on the Role of Zinc in Health and Disease. June 27, 1984, Isleworth, TIL Publications Ltd, 61-80
- **Jennings, IW,** Vitamins in Endocrine Metabolism. London, Heinemann, 1970.

- **Jervis, Ruth and Norman,** 'The Foresight Wholefood Cookbook', London, Roberts Publications, 1984.
- **Joffe, Justin M,** 'Influence of Drug Exposure on the Father on Perinatal Outcome', Clinics in Perinatology. Symposium of Pharmacology, 1979, 6(1), 21-36
- **Jones, Doris,** (1999), Fluoride, Damning new evidence, What Doctors Don't Tell You, Vol 9, No 12
- **Kamen, Betty and Si,** The Kamen Plan for Total Nutrition During Pregnancy, New York, Appleton-Century-Crofts, 1981, 24-30. This summarises a number of studies.
- **Kenton, Leslie and Susannah,** Raw Energy, London, Century, 1984, 32
- **Kirk, KM, Lyon, MF,** 'Induction of congenital malformations in the offspring of male mice treated with x-rays at premeiotic and post-meiotic stages', Mutation Research, 1984, 125,75-85
- **Klevay, Leslie M,** 'Hair as a Biopsy Material. Progress and Prospects'. Arch Intern Med. 1978, 138, 1127-1128.
- **Kostial, K, Kello, Dinko,** 'Bioavailability of lead in rats fed "human" diets' Bull Environ Comtam Toxicol, 1979, 21,312-314
- **Kupsinel, Roy,** 'Mercury Amalgam Toxicity. A major common denominator of Degenerative Disease' J Orthomolecular psychiatry, 13(4), 240-257
- **Labadarios, D,** 'Studies on The Effects of Drugs on Nutritional Status', 1975, Phd Thesis, University of Surrey
- **Lacranjan, I,** 'reproductive ability of workmen occupationally exposed to lead', Arch Environ Health, 1975, 20, 396-401
- **Laker, Martin,** 'On determining trace element levels in man: the uses of blood and hair'. Lancet, 1982, ii, 260-262.
- **Lappe, Mark,** 'Trace elements and the unborn: review and preliminary Implications for Policy' In Trace elements in Health. Ref 1, 237
- **Lees, Tony,** (2000), Toothpaste, A close brush with poison, What Doctors Don't Tell You, Vol 11, No 4
- **Lesser, Michael,** Nutrition and Vitamin Therapy, new York, Bantam, 1980.
- **Lester, Michael L, et al,** 'Protective Effects of Zinc and Calcium Against Heavy Metal Impairment of Children's Cognitive Function', Nutrition and Behaviour 1986, 2, 145-161
- **Lin-Fu, JS,** 'Vulnerability of children to lead exposure and toxicity" New Engl J Med, 1973, 289, 1229-1233
- **Little, Ruth E, Sing, Scharles F,** 'Father's Drinking and Infant Birth Weight: Report of an Association', Teratology, 1987, 36, 59-65
- **Lodge Rees, E,** 'Trace elements in pregnancy' Trace Elements in Health, Ed. J Rose, London, Butterworths, 1983, 262.
- **Lodge Rees, E,** 'Prevention versus problems in paediatric science', in The Next Generation, Anon, Witley, Surrey, Foresight, 1983, 2-12.

- **Lodge Rees, E,** 'The concept of preconceptual care;, Intern J. Environmental Studies, 1981, 17, 37-42.
- **Lodge Rees, Elizabeth,** 'Aluminium Toxicity as Indicated by Hair Analysis, J Orthomolecular Psychiatry, 1979, 8(1) 37-43
- **Mansfield, Peter, Monro, Jean,** Chemical Children, London, Century 1987, 31
- **Masefield, Jennifer,** 'Psychiatric Illness caused or exacerbated by Food Allergies', 1988 (unpublished paper)
- **Maugh, Thomas H,** 'Hair: A diagnostic Tool To Complement Blood Serum and Urine'. Science, 1978, 202, 1271-1273.
- **McCarrison, Sir Robert,** 'Nutrition and Health' McCarrison Society, 1984.
- **McDowall, ME,** 'OPCS Occupational Reproductive Epidemiology: The use of routinely collected statistics in England and Wales 1980-1982', studies on Medical and Population Subjects No. 50, London, HMSO 1985
- **McKie, Robin,** 'Cadmium in the diet poses health danger'. Sunday Times, 25 September 1983
- **Mercier, Chas,** 'Diet as a Factor in the Causation of Mental Disease', Lancet, 1916, i, 561.
- **Millstone, Erik, Abraham, John,** Additives. A Guide for Everyone, London, Penguin, 1988,11
- **Mohsen Moussa, Mohammed,** 'Caffeine and sperm motility', Fert Ster, 1983, 39, 845-848
- **Montagu, Ashley,**'Life Before Birth', New York, New American Library 196t, 23.
- **Moore, LS, Fleischman, Alan,** 'Subclinical lead toxicity' Orthomolecular psychiatry, 1975,4(1),61-70
- **Mortensen, Mary Lund et al,** 'Teratology and the Epidemiology of Birth Defects' In: Gabbe, Steven G et al, eds, Obstrics. Normal and Problem Pregnancies, New York, Churchill Livingstone, 1986, 183-210
- **Mortimer, G Rosen,** 'In the Beginning: Your Baby's Brain Before Birth', New York, New American Library, 1975, 25.
- **MRC Vitamin Study Group,** 'Prevention of neural tube defects: results of the Medical Research Council vitamin study', Lancet, 1991, 338, 131-7.
- **Needleman, H L et al,** 'Deficits in psychological and classroom performance of children with elevated dentine lead levels' New Eng J Med, 1979, 300, 689-696.
- **Neilson, Forrest H,** 'Nickel' in: Biochemistry of the Essential Ultratrace Elements, ed: Frieden, Earl. Plenum Publishing Corporation, 1984, 299
- **Nordstrom, S, et al,** 'Genetic defects in offspring of power-frequency workers'. Bioelectromagnetics, 1983, 4: 91
- **Nordstrom, S, et al,** 'Reproductive Hazards among workers at high-voltage systems. Bioelectromagnetics, 1981, 4, 91-101

- **Norwood, Christopher,** At Highest Risk, New York, McGraw Hill, 1980, 10-11
- **Norwood, Christopher,** At Highest Risk, New York, McGraw-Hill 1980, 190
- **Oberleas, Donald, Caldwell, Donald, Prasad, Ananda,** 'Trace Elements and Behaviour' Int Review Neurobiology Sup. 1972, 85
- **PAMA,** Vol 5, No 19, May 2002, Glass Ionomer Fillings, PAMA
- **Passwater, Richard A, and Cranton, Elmer M,** 'Trace Elements, Hair Analysis and Nutrition', New Canaan, Connecticut, Keats, 1983, 31-32
- **Passwater, Richard A, and Cranton, Elmer M,** Trace elements, Hair Analysis and Nutrition, new Canaan, NC, Keats, 1983.
- **Pfeiffer, Carl C,** 'Zinc and Other Micronutrients', New Canaan, Keats, 1978.
- **Pfeiffer, Carl D,** 'Mental and Elemental nutrients'. New Canaan, Connecticut, 1975, 169-170.
- **Pihl, RO, Parkes, M,** 'Hair element content in learning disabled children' Science, 1977, 198, 4214
- **Pottenger, FM Jr,** 'Pottenger's Cats'. La Mesa, CA, Price-Pottenger Nutrition Foundation, 1983.
- **Prentice, Thomson,** 'Anguish of the Sterile Husbands'. The Times, 20 April 1988,3.
- **Price, Weston A,** Nutrition and Physical Degeneration. La Mesa, CA, Price-Pottinger Foundation 1945, 397.
- **Reeves, John,** (2003), The Functions of Mycorrhiza, FORESIGHT Seminar
- **Report of the Board of Science and Education,** 'Diet, Nutrition and Health', British Medical Association, March 1986.
- **Rhodes, AJ,** Virus and Congenital Malformations. Papers and Discussions presented at the first International Conference on Congenital Malformations. Philadelphia-Lippincott, 1961.
- **Riggs, Alfred,** (2003), The Association of Earth Radiation & Other Fields with Specific Diseases, www.alfredriggs.com
- **Rosett, HL et al,** 'Patterns of Alcohol Consumption and Fetal Development', Obstet Gynecol, 1983, 61, 539-546
- **Rosso, P, Lederman, SA,** 'Nutrition in Pregnancy'. In: Proceedings of the 10th study group of the Royal College of Obstetricians and Gynaecologists, Ed. Campbell, D.M., Gillmer, M.D.G. September 1982, 115-130.
- **Rush, David, et al,** 'Diet in Pregnancy: A Randomised Controlled Trial of Nutritional Supplements', Birth Defects Original Article Series, Vol 16, No 3, New York, Alan R Liss Inc, 1980, 114.
- **Samarawickrama, Gervin,** 'Cadmium in animal and human health'. In: Trace elements and health. See ref 1, 37
- **Sandstead, Harry H,** 'Zinc: Essentiality for Brain Development and Function'. Nutrition Today 1984, November/December, 26-30

- **Saner, Gunay, Dagoglu and Ozden,** 'Hair manganese concentration in new-borns and their mothers', Am J clin Nut, 1985, 41, 1042-1044
- **Schauss, Alexander G,** Body Chemistry and Human Behaviour. Course: Oxford, 18 November 1986
- **Schell, Orville,** Modern Meat, New York, Random House, 1978, 176
- **Schroeder, Henry A,** The Trace Elements and Man, Old Greenwich, Devin-Adair, 1973, 152
- **Seidmann, Daniel S, Laor, Arie, et al,** 'Birth weight and intellectual performance in late adolescence' Obstet and Gynecol. 1992. 79:545-6
- **Shiva, Vandana,** (2000), Stolen Harvest, Zed Books
- **Shurygin, GI,** 'The psychogenic pathological development of personality in children and adolescents in families with fathers afflicted with alcoholism'. Zhur Nevropat I Psik, 1978, 78, 1566-1569 (Russian)
- **Singh, Nalini et al,** 'Neonatal lead intoxification in a prenatally exposed infant', J Paediatrics, 1978, 93(6), 1019-1021
- **Smith, GA,** 'Effects of maternal Undernutrition upon the newborn infant in Holland (1944-1945)' , J Pediatr, 1947, 30, 250-259.
- **Smith, JC et al,** 'Alterations in vitamin A metabolism during zinc deficiency and food and growth restriction'. J Nut, 1976, 106, 569-574.
- **Smith, JC et al,** 'Zinc: a trace element essential in vitamin A metabolism', Science, 1973, 181, 954-955.
- **Smithells, RW et al,** 'Further experience of vitamin supplementation for the prevention of neural tube defect recurrences', Lancet, 1983, I, 1027-1031.
- **Smithells, RW et al,** 'Possible prevention of neural tube defects by preconceptual vitamin supplementation' Lancet, 1980, I, 339-340
- **Socialist Countryside Group,** The Seed Scandal, Sevenoaks Socialist Countryside Group 1987
- **Sohler, Arthur et al,** 'Blood Lead Levels in Psychiatric Outpatients Reduced by Zinc And Vitamin C', J Orthomolecular Psychiatry, 1977, 6(3), 272-276
- **Soyka, LF, Joffe, JM,** 'Male mediated drug effects on offspring', Prog Clin Biol Res, 1980, 36, 49-66
- **Stenchever, MA, et al,** 'Chromosome Breakage in Users of Marijuana', Am J Obstet Gynecol, 1974, 118, 106-113
- **Stephens, Ian E,** (1987), Fluoridation - Mind Control of the Masses? The Dickinson Statement: A Mind-Boggling Thesis, Self Published
- **Storey, Christopher,** (2001), Cannabis Alert, The Lantern
- **Sullivan, Danny,** (1999), Ley Lines - A Comprehensive Guide to Alignments, Piatkus
- **Sutcliffe, Margaret, Schorah, Christopher J et al,** 'Prevention of neural tube defects', Lancet, 1993, 342, 1174
- **Thatcher, R et al,** 'Effects of low levels of cadmium and lead on cognitive functioning in children'. Arch Environ Health, 1982, 37(3), 159-166

- **Tokar, Brian,** (2001), Redesigning Life? The Worldwide Challenge to Genetic Engineering, Zed Books
- **Underwood, Eric J,** 'Trace Elements in Human and Animal Nutrition'. New York, Academic press, 1977, 152
- **Vogtmann, H,** 'The Quality of Agricultural Produce Originating From Different Systems of Cultivation'. Bristol, The Soil Association Ltd, 1979
- **Walker, Isobel,** 'The symptomless sex disease', Independent, 24 November 1987
- **Ward, NI et al,** 'Placental element Levels in Relation to Fetal Development for Obstetrically 'Normal' Births: A Study of 37 Elements. Evidence for Effects of Cadmium, Lead, and Zinc on Fetal Growth and Smoking as a Source of Cadmium', Int J Biosocial Res, 1987, 9(1), 63-81
- **Ward, NI, Brooks, RR,** 'Lead levels in sheep organs resulting from automotive exhausts' Environ Pollut, 1987, 17, 7-12
- **Ward, Neil I,** 'Preconceptual care questionnaire research project' 1990-92. Details from FORESIGHT
- **Wertheimer, N, Leeper, E,** Adverse effects on fetal development associated with sources of exposure to 60 Hz electric and magnetic fields (Abstract) 23r^d Hanford Life Sciences Symposium. Interaction of Biological Systems with Static and ELF Electric and Magnetic Fields, Richland, WA. 1984
- **Westrom, L,** 'Effect of acute pelvic infectious disease on fertility', Am J Obstet Gynecol, 1975, 121, 707-713
- **Wibberley, DG, et al,** 'Lead levels in human placentas from normal and malformed births' J Med Genetics, 1977, 14(5), 339-345
- **William, Roger J,** Nutrition Against Disease, New York, Bantam, 1973, 53.
- **Williams, Roger J,** Nutrition Against Disease, New York, Bantam 1971, 205
- **Williams, Roger J,** 'Biochemical individuality: the basis for the genotrophic concept', New York, Wiley, 1956.
- **Wynn, Arthur and Margaret,** 'Prevention of Handicap of Early Pregnancy Origin'. Today - Building Tomorrow: International Conference on Physical Disabilities, Montreal June 4-6, 1986, First Session.
- **Wynn, Margaret and Arthur,** 'Should Men and Women Limit Alcohol Consumption when hoping to have a baby', The Maternity Alliance (undated)
- **Yale, W et al,** 'Teachers' ratings of children's behaviour in relation to blood lead levels', Br J of Dev Psychology, 1985, 2, 295-306.
- **Young, Robin,** 'Pesticide found in a third of fresh fruit'. The Times, 16 April 1948
- **Yudkin, J,** Pure White and Deadly, London, Viking, 1986
- **Ziff,** The Toxic Time Bomb, Wellingborough, Thorsons, 1985

APPENDIX IV

RECOMMENDED READING LIST

- A BEGINNER'S INTRODUCTION TO TRACE MINERALS
  By E Di Cyon PhD

- A BEGINNER'S INTRODUCTION TO VITAMINS - the fundamental necessities for growth and maintenance of life
  By R A Passwater, PhD

- A MANUAL OF NATURAL FAMILY PLANNING
  By Dr Anna Flynn & Melissa Books

- AT HIGHEST RISK
  By Christopher Norwood

- CANDIDA ALBICANS - could yeast be your problem?
  By Leon Chaitnow

- EVALUATE YOUR OWN BIOCHEMICAL INDIVIDUALITY
  By Jeffrey Bland PhD

- FAMILY GUIDE TO HOMEOPATHY
  By Dr Andrew Lockie

- FATS THAT HEAL, FATS THAT KILL - Gerson Institute Healing Newsletter
  By Udo Erasmus

- FOODWATCH ALTERNATIVE COOKBOOK - wholefood recipes free of cow's milk wheat and chemical additives
  By Honour J Campbell

- FORESIGHT WHOLEFOOD COOKBOOK - for building healthy families
  By N & R Jarvis

- HOW TO GET WELL - proven effective solutions to your health problems
  By Paavo Aerola

- HYPERACTIVE CHILD
  By Belinda Barnes and Sally Bunday

- HYPOGLYCEMIA - a better approach
  By Paavo Aerola

- LET'S EAT RIGHT TO KEEP FIT
  By Adelle Davis

- MENTAL & ELEMENTAL NUTRIENTS - a physician's guide to nutrition & health care
  By Carl Pfeiffer MD, PhD

- NUTRITIONAL INFLUENCES OF ILLNESS - a source book of clinical research
  By Melvyn R Werbach, MD

- NUTRITION AND BEHAVIOUR - how what you eat affects what you do and can even prevent or promote delinquency
  By Alex Schauss, MS

- NUTRITION AND HEALTH
  By Sir Robert McCarrison

- NUTRITION AND PHYSICAL DEGENERATION - comparison of primitive and modern diets and their effects
  By Weston Price DDS

- PLANNING FOR A HEALTHY BABY
  By Belinda Barnes and Suzanne Gail Bradley

- POISONED HARVEST - a consumer's guide to pesticide use & abuse in the home as well as the wider environment
  By Christopher Robbins

- POTTINGER'S CATS - a study in nutrition
  By F M Pottinger Jnr, MD

- PREPARATION FOR PREGNANCY
  By Suzanne Gail Bradley and Nicholas Bennett

- PREVENTION OF HANDICAP OF EARLY PREGNANCY ORIGIN -some evidence of the value of good health before conception
  By M & A Wynn

- RAW ENERGY - eat your way to health
  By Leslie & Susannah Kenton

- THE CASE FOR PRECONCEPTUAL CARE OF MEN AND WOMEN
  By M&A Wynn

- THE DRIVING FORCE - food, evolution and the future
  By Michael Crawford & David Marsh

- THE FOOD ALLERGY HANDBOOK - a working doctor's self-help guide to new medical discoveries
  By Dr Keith Mumby

- THE LIVING SOIL & THE HAUGHLEY EXPERIMENT - evidence of the importance to human health of soil vitality
  By E B Balfour

- THE NATURAL WAY TO BETTER BABIES
  By Francesca Naish & Janette Roberts

- THE TRACE ELEMENTS & MAN
  By Henry Schroeder, MD

- THE VITAMIN BIBLE - how the right vitamins and minerals can revolutionise your life
  By Earl Mindell

- THE WHOLE HEALTH GUIDE TO ELEMENTAL HEALTH
  By Patrick Holford

- TRACE ELEMENTS, HAIR ANALYSIS & NUTRITION
  By R Passwater PhD & E M Cranton MD

- TRACE ELEMENTS IN HUMAN AND ANIMAL NUTRITION
  By E J Underwood

- YOUR HOME, YOUR HEALTH AND WELLBEING
  By WJ Rea,MD

- VITAMINS IN ENDOCRINE METABOLISM
  By Isobel Jennings, MRCVS

- ZINC AND OTHER MICRONUTRIENTS
  By Carl Pfeiffer MD, PhD

APPENDIX V

USEFUL ADDRESSES

- Abel & Cole, Organic Food (London Area),
  Unit 29-30, MGI Estates, Milkwood Road, London, SE24 OJE
  (0800 376 4040) (020 7737 3648)

- Action Against Allergy, Mrs Patricia Schooling,
  24/26 High Street, Hampton Hill, Middlesex, TW12 1PD
  (020 8943 4244)

- Ainsworth Homeopathic Chemist, 38 New Cavendish Street,
  London, S1M 7LH (020 7935 5330)

- ASH (Association for Smoking & Health) (020 7935 3519)

- Association for Homeopathic Medicine, 21 Leaze Park Road,
  Newcastle-upon-Tyne, NE1 4PE

- Association of General Practitioners of Natural Medicine,
  38 Nigel House, Portpool Lane, London, EC1N 7UR
  (020 7405 2781)

- Billings Method, 12 Eastwood, Three Bridges Road, Crawley,
  W Sussex. (01293 21754)

- British Association of Holistic Health, 179 Gloucester Place,
  London, NW1 6DX (0207 262 5299)

- British Organic Farmers Association, Leggatts Park,
  Potters Bar, Herts, EN6 1NZ

- British Society for Allergy & Environmental Medicine,
  PO Box 7, Knighton, Powys, LD7 1WZ (0906 302 0010)

- British Society for Nutritional Medicine, PO Box 3AP,
  London W1A 3AP

- CMAC NFP Services, 1 Blythe Mews, Blythe Road, London, W14 0NW

- Ecology Building Society, 8 Main Street, Cross Hills, Keighley, West Yorkshire, BD20 8TD (01535 35933)

- Eco-Paints, Unit 34, Heysham Business Park, Middleton Road, Heysham, Lancs, LA3 3PP.

- Ecover, Chatham Court Farm, Steyning, Sussex

- Electromagnetic pollution/Radiation (where to find help)

  Dr Patrick MacManaway, Whole Earth Geomancy, Westbank Natural Health Centre, Strathmiglo, Fife, Scotland, KY14 7QP (01337 868945)

  Dr Roger Coghill, Coghill Research Laboratory, Kermenez Lower Race, Pontypool, S.Wales NP4 5UH. (01495 752122 office hours)

  Mr Roy Riggs (home visits) Electromagnetic and Geopathic Energy Surveyor, 25 Coleridge St, Hove, Sussex, BN3 5AB (01273 732523) (roy-riggs@ntlworld.com)

- Environmental Air Systems, Martin Wells, Sandyhill Cottage, Sandy Land, Rushmore, Tilford, Surrey, GU10 2ET

- Ewes' Milk, The Brimar Flock, Downe House Farm, Sessay, Thirsk, North Yorkshire (01845 401221)

- FACT, (Food Additives Campaign Team), 25 Horsell Road, London, N5 1XL (020 7633 8939)

- Fertility Trust, 218 Heathwood Road, Heath, Cardiff, CF4 4BS

- Food Commission, Third Floor, 5/11 Worship Street, London, EC2A 2BH

- FORESIGHT, 28 The Paddock, Godalming, Surrey, GU7 1XD (01483 427839)

- FORESIGHT Laboratory, Unit 6, Brocklands Farm, West Meon, Hants (01730 829861) (Fax 01730 829862)

- FORESIGHT Resource Centre, Mead House, Ladymead Estate, Alfold Road, Godalming, Surrey (01483 548071) (Fax 01483 548070)

- Freshwater Filters, Carlton House, Aylmer Road, Leytonstone, E11 3AD

- Friends of the Earth, 26-28 Underwood Street, London, N1 7JQ (020 7490 1556)

- Goats' Milk, Vita Care, (0191 383 0646)

- Good Gardeners Association, Pinetum Lodge, Churcham, Gloucester, GL2 8AD (01594 861196)

- Greenlink, (Research into Environmental Factors) 9 Clairmont Road, Lexton Heath, Colchester, Essex, CO3 SBE (01206 46902)

- Greenpeace, Canonbury Villas, London, N1 2PE (020 7865 8100)

- Healthy House, Cold Harbour, Ruscombe, Stroud, Glos, GL6 6DA (01453 752216)

- Henry Doubleday Research Association, (Organic Gardening) Ryton on Dunsmore, Coventry, CV8 3LG (01203 303517)

- Hockeys (Organic Meat), Newton Farm, South Gorley, Fordingbridge, Hants, (01425 625542)

- ION, Blades Court, Deodar Road, Putney, SW15 (020 8877 9980)

- Journal of Alternative & Complementary Medicine (020 7385 0012)

- Lifestyle (Gluten Free Bread and other products), Centenary Business Park, Station Road, Henley on Thames, Oxon, RG9 1DS (01491 411 767)

- London Hazards Centre, Hampstead Town Hall, 213 Haverstock Hill, NW3 4QP (020 7794 5999)

- National Childbirth Trust, Alexandra House, Oldham Terrace, Acton, London, W3 7NH (020 8992 8637)

- Organic Food Service, Ashe, Churston Ferrers, Brixham, Devon

- Organic Growers' Association, Aeron Park, Llangietho, Dyfed

- Parascope Microbiology Laboratory, Chapel Allerston Hospital, Chapeltown Road, Leeds, LS7 4SA (0113 3924657)

- PEX, Pesticide Trust, Eurolink House, 49 Effra Road, London, SW12 1BZ (020 7274 8895)

- Plasketts Nutritional Medical College, Three Quions House, Launceston, Cornwall, PL15 8SJ (01566 86301)

- Plastic Pipes (Hepworth) (01226 763561)

- Plastic Pipes Association (0121 236 1866)

- Society for the Promotion of Nutritional Therapy, PO Box 47, Heathfield, East Sussex, TN21 8ZX (01435 867007)

- Society of Homeopaths, 101 Sebastian Avenue, Shenfield, Brentwood, Essex.

- Soil Association, Bristol House, 40-56 Victoria Street, Bristol, BN1 6BY (01179 290661)

- The Raworth College of Nutrition, South Street, Dorking, Surrey (01360 742150)

- What Doctors Don't Tell You, The Informed Parent, and "Proof", Satellite House, 2 Salisbury Road, London, SW19 4EZ (0800 146054)

INDEX

217